Gay Personality and Sexual Labeling

T0314617

Gay Personality
and
Sexual Labeling

Edited by
John P. De Cecco

Gay Personality and Sexual Labeling was originally published in 1984 by The Haworth Press, Inc., under the title *Bisexual and Homosexual Identities: Critical Clinical Issues.* It has also been published as *Journal of Homosexuality,* Volume 9, Number 4, Summer 1984.

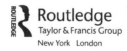

Routledge
Taylor & Francis Group
New York London

First published by

Harrington Park Press, Inc. is a Subsidiary of The Haworth Press, Inc., 12 West 32 Street, New York, New York 10001.

This edition published 2012 by Routledge

Routledge   Routledge
Taylor & Francis Group   Taylor & Francis Group
711 Third Avenue   27 Church Road
New York, NY 10017   Hove, East Sussex BN3 2FA

Gay Personality and Sexual Labeling was originally published in 1984 by The Haworth Press, Inc. under the title *Bisexual and Homosexual Identities: Critical Clinical Issues*. It has also been published as *Journal of Homosexuality*, Volume 9, Number 4, Summer 1984.

Library of Congress Cataloging in Publication Data

Bisexual and homosexual identities, critical clinical issues.
    Gay personality and sexual labeling.

    Reprint. Originally published: Bisexual and homosexual identities, critical clinical issues. New York : Haworth Press, c1984.
    Includes bibliographical references and index.
    1. Homosexuality—Addresses, essays, lectures. 2. Bisexuality—Addresses, essays, lectures. 3. Sex (Psychology)—Addresses, essays, lectures. 4. Identity (Psychology)—Addresses, essays, lectures. I. De Cecco, John. II. Title.
HQ76.25.B565   1985   306.7'65   84-22578
ISBN 0-918393-01-9 (pbk.)

CONTENTS

BOOK REVIEWS

The *Journal of Homosexuality* is devoted to theoretical, empirical, and historical research on homosexuality, heterosexuality, sexual identity, social sex roles, and the sexual relationships of both men and women. It was created to serve the allied disciplinary and professional groups represented by psychology, sociology, history, anthropology, biology, medicine, the humanities, and law. Its purposes are:

   a) to bring together, within one contemporary scholarly journal, theoretical, empirical, and historical research on human sexuality, particularly sexual identity;
   b) to serve as a forum for scholarly research of heuristic value for the understanding of human sexuality, based not only in the more traditional social or biological sciences, but also in literature, history and philosophy;
   c) to explore the political, social, and moral implications of research on human sexuality for professionals, clinicians, social scientists, and scholars in a wide variety of disciplines and settings.

EDITOR

JOHN P. De CECCO, PhD, *Professor of Psychology and Director, Center for Research and Education in Sexuality (CERES), San Francisco State University*

MANUSCRIPT EDITOR

WENDELL RICKETTS, *Center for Research and Education in Sexuality*

ASSOCIATE EDITORS

STUART KELLOGG, MONIKA KEHOE, and MICHAEL G. SHIVELY, *Center for Research and Education in Sexuality*

FOUNDING EDITOR

CHARLES SILVERSTEIN, *Institute for Human Identity, New York City*

EDITORIAL BOARD

ROGER AUSTEN, *Teaching Fellow, University of Southern California, Los Angeles*
ALAN BELL, PhD, *Department of Counseling, Indiana University*
PHILIP W. BLUMSTEIN, PhD, *Associate Professor of Sociology, University of Washington*
VERN L. BULLOUGH, PhD, *Dean, Faculty of Natural and Social Sciences, State University of New York College, Buffalo*
ELI COLEMAN, PhD, *Assistant Professor and Coordinator of Clinical Services, Program in Human Sexuality, University of Minnesota*
LOUIE CREW, PhD, *Associate Professor of English, University of Wisconsin, Stevens Point*
LOUIS CROMPTON, PhD, *Professor of English, University of Nebraska, Lincoln*
MARTIN DANNECKER, PhD, *Abteilung für Sexualwissenschaft, Klinikum der Johann Wolfgang Goethe Universität, Frankfurt am Main, West Germany*
JOSHUA DRESSLER, JD, *Professor of Law, Wayne State University Law School*
LILLIAN FADERMAN, PhD, *Professor of English, California State University, Fresno*
BYRNE R. S. FONE, PhD, *Associate Professor of English, The City College, City University of New York*
JOHN GAGNON, PhD, *Professor of Sociology, State University of New York at Stony Brook*
JOHN GONSIOREK, PhD, *Clinical Psychologist, Twin Cities Therapy Clinic, Minneapolis, Minnesota; Clinical Assistant Professor, Department of Psychology, University of Minnesota*
ERWIN HAEBERLE, PhD, *Director of Historical Research, Institute for the Advanced Study of Human Sexuality, San Francisco*

RICHARD HALL, MA, *Writer, New York City*

JOEL D. HENCKEN, MA, *Private Practice, Boston; PhD Candidate in Clinical Psychology, University of Michigan*

EVELYN HOOKER, PhD, *Retired Research Professor, Psychology Department, University of California, Los Angeles*

RICHARD J. HOFFMAN, PhD, *Associate Professor, Department of History, San Francisco State University*

FRED KLEIN, MD, *Clinical Institute for Human Relationships, San Diego*

MARY RIEGE LANER, PhD, *Associate Professor of Sociology, Arizona State University, Tempe*

ELLEN LEWIN, PhD, *Medical Anthropology Program, University of San Francisco*

DON LILES, MA, *Instructor in English, City College of San Francisco*

A. P. MACDONALD, JR., PhD, *Acting Director and Associate Professor, Center for the Family, University of Massachusetts, Amherst*

WILLIAM F. OWEN, MD, *Private Practice, San Francisco*

L. ANNE PEPLAU, PhD, *Associate Professor of Psychology, University of California, Los Angeles*

KENNETH PLUMMER, PhD, *Department of Sociology, University of Essex, England*

SHARON RAPHAEL, PhD, *Associate Professor of Sociology, California State University, Dominguez-Hills*

KENNETH READ, PhD, *Professor of Anthropology, University of Washington, Seattle*

MICHAEL ROSS, PhD, *Senior Demonstrator in Psychiatry, The Flinders University of South Australia, Adelaide, Australia*

DOROTHY SEIDEN, PhD, *Professor, Department of Home Economics, San Francisco State University*

G. WILLIAM SKINNER, PhD, *Professor of Anthropology, Stanford University*

RICHARD W. SMITH, PhD, *Professor of Psychology, California State University, Northridge*

JOHN P. SPIEGEL, MD, *Director, Training Program in Ethnicity and Mental Health, Brandeis University; Current President, American Academy of Psychoanalysis*

FREDERICK SUPPE, PhD, *Chair, Committee on the History and Philosophy of Science, University of Maryland, College Park*

JOHN UNGARETTI, MA, *Classics; MA, Literature; San Francisco*

JEFFREY WEEKS, PhD, *Research Fellow, Department of Sociology, University of Essex, England*

JAMES WEINRICH, PhD, *Psychiatry and Behavioral Sciences, Johns Hopkins University*

JACK WIENER, MSW, *Retired, National Institute of Mental Health, Bethesda, Maryland*

DEBORAH WOLF, PhD, *Institute for the Study of Social Change, University of California, Berkeley*

WAYNE S. WOODEN, PhD, *Assistant Professor, Behavioral Science, California State Polytechnic University, Pomona*

Foreword

The present issue follows on the heels of the two previous issues (numbers 2 and 3) in this volume of the *Journal,* entitled the *Bisexual and Homosexual Identities: Critical Theoretical Issues.* Those numbers were devoted to an examination of the idea of sexual identity as it occurs within historical, bisexual, homosexual, and biological contexts in the discourse on sexual identity. The present issue continues the discussion of sexual identity, now within a clinical context. "Clinical context" has been broadly defined to include depth psychology, diagnostic classification, therapy, and psychomedical research on the hormonal basis of homosexuality.

In the articles which follow, Martin Dannecker, within the framework of a reformulated depth psychology, proposes a conception of the homosexual identity as a psychical entity developmentally distinct from the heterosexual identity. Beyond the homosexual identity, Fred Suppe and Charles Silverstein suggest there is a long list of sexual identities, equally venerable in the professional annals of perversion, which remain to be depathologized by psychiatry. Along with "ego-dystonic homosexuality," they argue that the paraphilias now listed in the diagnostic manuals are little more than invocations of moral judgments and endorsements of prevailing moral codes.

As clinicians, John Hart and Joel Hencken explore the therapeutic implications of labels. Hart reminds therapists that the success of their enterprise hinges on the beliefs of their clients about sexual identity and not their own theoretical predilections. Hencken adumbrates the many ways in which clients can deceive themselves and others about the meaning of their homosexual behavior—engaging in the behavior while avoiding the homosexual label.

The search for the biological basis for the homosexual orientation has been carried on as a branch of clinical medicine, frequently under the auspices of psychiatry. In a comprehensive review of the literature, Wendell Ricketts points out the theoretical and methodological deficiencies in the research and the implicit moral beliefs and cultural prejudices that apparently inhere in what is purportedly a scientific enterprise in biology and medicine.

The editor gratefully acknowledges the thoughtful and persuasive contributions of the authors and the assistance of Norman C. Hopper, the new manuscript editor, and the new *Journal* secretaries, Mary M. Walsh and Jocelyn Sison.

John P. De Cecco, PhD
Editor

Gay Personality
and
Sexual Labeling

Towards a Theory of Homosexuality: Socio-Historical Perspectives

Martin Dannecker, PhD

J. W. Goethe-Universität

Historical studies generally agree that a far-reaching change has taken place in social attitudes toward homosexuality, although they disagree as to when this change occurred. The change resulted from a scientific discourse which extended a unitary sexuality into sexualities, a process that Michel Foucault (1978) described so strikingly as the "implantation of perversions." He was referring to the significant increase in discussions of the peripheral forms of sexuality since the 19th century, those which are termed "deviant" in the language of modern sociology. The importance these forms of sexuality were given is evident in the fact that they became a separate field of research: "psychopathia sexualis." Sexually deviant behavior was classified as unnatural, pathological, or anti-social. This branding, of course, did not stop the peripheral sexualities from preoccupying social consciousness and becoming possible, however dangerous, behaviors.

In contrast to other authors, Foucault (1978) located this change in attitudes toward homosexuality in the 19th century, when the growing medical, educational, and psychological scientization of sexuality occurred. Foucault (1978) writes: "The nineteenth-century homosexual became a personage, a past, a case history and a childhood, in addition to being a type of life, a life form, and a morphology, with an indiscreet anatomy and possibly a mysterious physiology" (p. 43).

The homosexual personality which began to emerge in scientific texts was by no means widely welcomed. The homosexual was introduced into social consciousness *persona non grata.* However, just as a wider public

Dr. Dannecker obtained his doctoral degree in social psychology. He presently teaches in Abteilung für Sexualwissenschaft (Department of Sexology) at Frankfurt University. He is the author of *Theories of Homosexuality* (1978) and the script writer for Rosa von Praunheim's film *It's Not the Homosexual That's Perverted, But the Society in Which He Lives.* This paper was read at the 8th Annual Meeting of the International Academy of Sex Research, August 22-26, 1982, Copenhagen. Requests for reprints should be addressed to the author, Klinikum der J. W. Goethe-Universität, Abteilung für Sexualwissenschaft, Theodor-Stern-Kai 7, 6000 Frankfurt am Main 70, Federal Republic of Germany.

frequently first learns of the existence of a person when that person is declared *persona non grata* by the government, so it was that the homosexual first came to public notice through scandalization.

However, the scientific texts on homosexuality have not been able to give the newly created, separate homosexual figure personal substance. Their description of the characteristics of homosexuals have been vague and contradictory. Scarcely has a trait been defined by one author as typical for homosexuals than another responds by asserting that the same trait can also be observed in heterosexuals. This protracted dispute cannot be resolved by isolating personal characteristics, since the picture of a homosexual as a person is more than the sum of the parts used to form this picture.

Sex research in its earliest days did little more to validate its conception of homosexuality than to invoke the old religious ethics. What religious ethics formerly viewed as morally proscribed was treated by sex research as organically or mentally inferior. This is why sex research was caught up for a long time in the old belief that sexuality always meant heterosexuality.

The classification by Krafft-Ebing and his precursors of homosexuality as psychopathological, long remained the last word in established science, although the symptoms assumed to justify this classification have changed in the course of time. Nevertheless, the general classification of homosexuality as pathological remained unchanged for several decades.

Let us bear in mind the following: The more homosexuality was viewed as a distinct pathology, the more the conception of the homosexual as a special kind of person was consolidated. The conception of the homosexual as a person became a central idea in the older texts on homosexuality.

Whereas in the established scientific dispute the homosexual was recognized as a person only when labeled pathological, there developed a divergent approach in fringe circles revolving around Carl Heinrich Ulrichs, Magnus Hirschfeld, and Iwan Bloch. These authors also considered homosexuals to be distinct entities, although their differentiation was not based on pathology. In Ulrichs' (1864/1978) opinion there existed a separate class of congenital homosexuals, whom he called "urnings." By congenital he meant "sexual, organic, and mental inheritance . . . inheritance such as Dionians (or heterosexuals) receive in their sexual love for women and vice versa" (p. 4). This line of thought led to Magnus Hirschfeld's famous classification of homosexuals as the "third sex."

This change in the conception of homosexuality was commented on by Foucault (1978): "Homosexuality appeared as one of the forms of sexuality when it was put down from the practice of sodomy onto a kind of interior androgyny, a hermaphroditism of the soul." Foucault's position comes very close to that taken by the labeling approach in sociology, which also claims that the idea of a distinct homosexual personality is an artifact of social reaction to homosexual behavior.[1]

Foucault takes an extremely critical attitude towards the historical turning-point in social reaction toward homosexuality. He seems convinced not only that the scientific discourse on homosexuality in medicine, psychology, and sexual science actually created the homosexual figure, but also that this very discourse has negatively transformed the homosexual. Directly after the sentence quoted above he continues with the words: "The sodomite had been a temporary aberration; the homosexual was now a species."[2]

Although I share Foucault's opinion that a change in social reaction toward homosexuality has taken place, my evaluation of the effects it has had on homosexuals differs from his. He creates the impression that the scientific debate has put something fundamentally new on the historical map. This does not seem plausible to me. To be sure, the manner in which a phenomenon is discussed will not fail to have an influence on it, since speech influences perceptions and reactions. However, it is problematical as to how and with what profundity discourse fathoms and transforms a phenomenon. Foucault and, even more, the sociologists who have adopted the labeling approach, have overestimated the effect of both the discourse and social definitions on homosexuality as a phenomenon in its own right.

We know only a few details of behavior of those who were called sodomites in the legal texts of past centuries. It may well be that this behavior was as transitory and fortuitous as Foucault would have us believe. On the other hand, it could be that sodomites were persons essentially similar to the modern homosexual. We know as little about the possible structural difference between a sodomite and a heterosexual of the 17th century as we do about the possible structural similarities between a homosexual of our day and the sodomite of previous centuries. The reason we know so little is simply because neither medicine nor any other department of science had formulated human sexuality as a field of inquiry.

The concept of homosexuality went no further than the concept of a sexual act. This conceptualization placed homosexual conduct in a criminal category. An important penal code of the 16th century (the *Constitutio Criminalis Bambergensis*) states the following: "Whensoever an unchaste act is committed by a person with an animal, by a man with a man, or by a woman with a woman, he has forfeited his life and shall be condemned to death by fire as is common custom" (G. Bleibtreu-Ehrenberg, 1978, p. 297). The concept of the act on which this penal code is based completely precludes any understanding of the individual actor.

In contrast, sexology, medicine, and psychology have been interested in deep comprehensive understanding of the phenomenon of homosexuality. However poorly this task was accomplished, "the will to understand" formed the central motive of the scientific discourse.

Compared with the previous social reactions to homosexual conduct, the discourse represents progress even if it is motivated by the intention to establish more effective control by means of deeper knowledge. Such control aimed at by society or, as Foucault would say, by power, could only be implemented by loosening the previously harsh repression. Nowhere is this loosening of control more evident than in the history of homosexuality.

Before the 19th century, when a homosexual act was made public the person accused was given the death sentence. It was neither possible nor necessary in the light of the prevailing historical circumstances to gain knowledge about or even an understanding of the essence of the accused party. This deeper understanding requires a way of dealing with the homosexual act that allows for a delay between its public revelation and the execution of the accused. During this delay homosexuality can possibly be examined. The accused can step forward and speak. However, the moment he or she has spoken, homosexuality is given expression as a possible way of life. Its formerly secret existence becomes public. Even if the phenomenon or its embodiment were eliminated, it nonetheless would have indelibly expressed itself as one possible form of life.

The historical change which transformed the simple homosexual act into a special kind of person, I consider an important moment in historical progress and one of the main achievements of the theory of homosexuals to assume an identity of their own. It was one of the decisive conditions for being able to take up the fight against antihomosexual repression.

It is, consequently, anything but a coincidence that the first homosexual rights movement gathered round the theorist who recognized homosexuality not only as innate but also as indelible: Magnus Hirschfeld and the "Wissenschaftlich Humanitäre Komitee." For all that, Hirschfeld managed only to biologize homosexuals by ignoring the difference between the categories "homosexuality" and "homosexual." Thus, despite his constant protestations to the contrary, the actual object of Hirschfeld's research was not homosexuality. His interests were centered on the particular form of homosexuality displayed by the homosexual individuals of his time—what I have called "manifest homosexuality" (Dannecker, 1978).

Sigmund Freud (1905-1953) raised serious objection to this reductionism and to the biological separation of homosexuals it implied in a footnote added to his *Three Essays on the Theory of Sexuality.* Freud claimed that all human beings are capable of choosing an object of their own sex and have in fact already done so in their unconscious. He set for research the task of elucidating the exclusive sexual interest felt by men for women. Freud's objection should by no means be interpreted as the intention to eradicate all differences between homosexuals and heterosexuals. His criticism is levelled at biologizing homosexuals and thus understating the theoretical and practical problems of research on homosexuality.

Freud expressly adhered to the belief in the common origin of manifest homosexuality and heterosexuality. Moreover, he did not allow himself to be deluded by differences that existed between manifest homosexuals and manifest heterosexuals. There are differences between homosexuals and heterosexuals that are apparent and not limited to social behavior but point to differences in general development of personality. Such differences are still not due to qualitatively different determinants. Freud's (1905/1953) comment was: "The differences in the end-products may be of a qualitative nature, but analysis shows that the differences between their determinants are only quantitative" (p. 57). Let us bear in mind that in Freud's view there was no distinct homosexual nature. He did, however, recognize differences in personality of an order that he called qualitative.

Alfred Kinsey and his associates (1948) need to dispose of the idea of the homosexual as a unique personality. They refused to use the term "the homosexual," which implies differences, instead referring to individuals "who have had certain amounts of heterosexual experience and certain amounts of homosexual experience" (p. 617).

Kinsey and his associates were not content merely to describe quantitative conditions; they also made an attempt to explain them. They were, in effect, inspired by the same question that had sparked the old theories of etiology. The question is: How can it happen that some individuals develop no homosexual forms of behavior, some partially do, while others are exclusively homosexual. About the exclusively homosexual, Kinsey, Pomeroy, and Martin (1948) wrote:

> One of the factors that materially contributes to the development of exclusively homosexual histories is the ostracism which society imposes upon one who is discovered to have perhaps no more than a lone experience. The high school boy is likely to be expelled from school and, if it is in a small town, he is almost certainly to be driven from the community. His chances of making heterosexual contacts are tremendously reduced after the public disclosure, and he is forced into the company of other homosexual individuals among whom he finally develops an exclusively homosexual pattern for himself. (p. 663)

This formulation shows that the Kinsey group was clearly a precursor of the labeling approach. Similarly, they conceived homosexuality as a diffuse experience that any person was capable of. Their explanation for strikingly different patterns was sought in external conditions, that is, in conditions that are more or less fortuitous but decisively determine sexual orientation. In the Kinseyian conception the personality differences that exist before the first sexual experiences are ignored. Any perceived differences were attributed to factors that influenced the individual after the first homosexual encounter.

Authors who take a similar, even if more sophisticated viewpoint, revert to Freud's concept of "polymorphous perversity" and constitutional bisexuality to support the premise that homosexuality is a diffuse experience any person can have. This was not Freud's position. Freud was, after all, a psychoanalyst, and the early childhood years were determinative of sexual development. In childhood the fundamental sexual openness that Freud postulated becomes structured. This is the price paid for growing up. In early childhood, sexuality assumes a form; that is, the diffuse instinct acquires a destiny. Whether it assumes the heterosexual or homosexual form, it will become an integral part of the person so that the individual is no longer able to dispose of it at will. The individual will, therefore, be restricted in the range of sexual choices. This means, however, that experiences later on in life are dependent not only on external circumstances and events but also inner structure, i.e., on the specific personality that is linked to particular sexual preferences, aversions, anxieties, and fixations.

My thesis is that a sexual disposition is acquired in early childhood which determines adult behavior. This disposition does not determine future behavior in all its details. Reading the etiological theories of homosexuality, one often has the impression that behavior is predetermined in every respect. There is an inadequate analysis in etiological theories of the social constraints that one is subject to as an adolescent or adult. Labeling theory contains a just response to the inadequate understanding in the etiological theories of the behavior of social minorities.

But while etiological theories of homosexuality placed a biased emphasis on the restrictions and constraints that stem from the psychological system and understated the never-ending social forces that burden individuals, the sociological approach understated the inner personality factors. Symbolic interactionism, which is the basis for the labeling approach, holds (Plummer, 1981) that: "Initially our experiences are much more random, unstructured and uncrystallized than we choose to believe, and that it is through the definitional process that this randomness becomes channelled into stable sexual identities" (p. 69).

Present research on homosexuality is inhibited by the fact that it handles the psychological and sociological perspectives as competing models and thus perpetuates their dogmatically constricted validity. Consequently, the labeling approach does not consider either inner constraints or the insight to be gained from clinical research. The psychological perspective telescopes all factors into a person's inner being so as to be able to treat homosexuality as an illness. Psychological research, however, considers the labeling approach to be very superficial since its only concern is for the social aspects of a person and not deeper personal layers. Critics of the labeling approach not unjustly assert that it relinguishes the very idea of the person.

If, however, recent assertions are true that there is evidence for both psychological and sociological models, then the present theoretical dilemma would be resolved. Evidence in support of both models derives from the results of empirical investigations that indicate, on one hand, "change of identities," and demonstrate, on the other, an early and stable "homosexual identity." The dilemma stems less from the empirical findings than in the way they are interpreted, particularly in the use made of the concept of identity. There is, of course, a considerable difference between having a homosexual identity and having a homosexual praxis. Large numbers of men engage in homosexual behavior for long periods of time without acquiring the slightest traces of homosexual identity.

However, I do not believe that the concept of identity can be applied to those empirical studies on adult homosexuals that show that many knew at a very early age that they were homosexual. Identity is acquired relatively late in life. Once it has established itself, the person retrospectively reconstructs his biography in its light. There is certainly no doubt that many homosexuals felt in early childhood that they were different. This early feeling of being different, however, should not be confused with having acquired a homosexual identity. This early sense of difference is a diffuse, often agonizing, feeling that has no name. Although it is the early expression of distinct psychic structure, the feeling is not yet integrated with a conscious homosexual identity.

In a recently published discussion (Plummer, 1981), leading proponents of the labeling perspectives feared their position might be jeopardized by homosexuals reporting that they felt as children that they were different.[3] The results of the study by Bell, Weinberg, and Smith (1981) would probably deepen these fears. This study compared homosexual men and women with their heterosexual counterparts for "gender conformity." The study showed decisive differences between the two groups and that, long before a homosexual becomes a social personality, he or she differs from the heterosexual. The authors summarized these results by pointing out that the ultimate preference for homosexuality is already reflected or expressed in the first traces of a distinct behavior, although the preference is by no means determined by the differences in behavior. Despite these results we should not overestimate the differences in personality structure. There is, of course, no direct connection between these early signs of structural differences and the homosexual identity acquired later. Homosexual identity is only established in the confrontation with reality. This is evident in the fact that the structural differences between homosexuals and heterosexuals lead to differing social experiences very early on. The contrasting experiences not only consolidate the already existing differences in personality structure but also reshape it.

Why should homosexuals not be different from the others in the deeper layers of personality? If they were not, then they would not have become homosexuals. A homosexual does indeed go through a specific development at a very early stage of socialization. Since this development does not take place in a vacuum but within a specific social context, the ultimate form it assumes is also dependent on social reaction to its development. In childhood these differences are not dealt with in terms of homosexuality or heterosexuality, but in terms of gender role. A young boy is judged, for example, to be less athletic or manly.

In conclusion, the individual homosexual is a product of the social environment he or she encounters when the homosexual orientation begins to emerge. Only in this regard is the individual *made* a homosexual. However, only that person becomes a homosexual whose personal structure allows this possibility. In this regard, an individual *is* a homosexual.

REFERENCE NOTES

1. Consequently it is not a great surprise that Kenneth Plummer (1981) chose the Foucault excerpt from which I took the sentence quoted above as a motto for his book, "The Making of the Modern Homosexual." In the English translation of Foucault's (1978) book, "transposed" is used to translate the original French word "rabattre." The word "transposed" is far too neutral in this context. The meaning of the verb "rabattre" is more precisely rendered in English by "to put down" rather than by "to transpose."

2. The English translation adds the adjective "temporary" to the French version. This addition renders Foucault's intention precisely. Being a sympathizer of a somewhat anarchustic life style, Foucault's intention was to distinguish between the chance character of the sodomite and the notion of the "homosexual" in the scientific discourse.

3. I am referring to Mary McIntosh, Kenneth Plummer, and Jeffrey Weeks and their discussion about "the homosexual role" (Plummer, 1981, pp. 44-49).

REFERENCES

Bell, A. P., Weinberg, M., & Smith, S. K. (1981). *Sexual preference: A study of development among men and women.* Indianapolis, IN: University of Indiana Press.

Bleibtreu-Ehrenberg, G. (1978). *Tabu homosexualität.* Frankfurt a.M.: Fischer.

Dannecker, M. (1981). *Theories of homosexuality.* London: Gay Men's Press. (Originally published in German in 1978)

Foucault, M. (1978). *The history of sexuality, vol. 1: An introduction.* (R. Hurley, trans.) New York: Random House.

Freud, S. (1953). *Three essays on the theory of sexuality.* In J. Strachey (Trans., Ed.,), *The standard editions of the complete psychological works of Sigmund Freud. Vol. VII.* London: The Hogarth press. (Originally published, 1905)

Kinsey, A., Pomeroy, W., & Martin, C. (1948). *Sexual behavior in the human male.* Philadelphia: W. B. Saunders.

Plummer, K. (Ed.) (1981). *The making of the modern homosexual.* London: Hutchinson.

Ulrichs, C. H. (1978). *Vindx.* Los Angeles: Urania Manuscripts. (Originally published in German in 1864 under the pseudonym "Numa Numantius")

Classifying Sexual Disorders:
The *Diagnostic and Statistical Manual*
of the American Psychiatric Association

Frederick Suppe, PhD

University of Maryland

ABSTRACT. The objectivity of the classification of sexual disorders in the third edition of the *Diagnostic and Statistical Manual* (DSM-III) of the American Psychiatric Association is explored via a critical examination of (1) the replacement of homosexuality per se by ego-dystonic homosexuality, (2) DSM's working concept of a mental disorder, (3) the notion of a paraphilia, (4) components of sexual identity, and (5) the literature on variant sexual behaviors. It is argued that (a) the same criteria that led to the removal of homosexuality *per se* as a mental disorder require the removal of all the paraphilias *per se*, (b) there is no empirical warrant to justify their continued inclusion, and (c) while there is legitimacy for a generalized ego-dystonic category, such ego-dystonias are only incidentally sexual. It is suggested that the present classification of sexual disorders is merely the codification of social mores.

Health consists in having the same diseases as one's neighbors.
— Quentin Crisp, *The Naked Civil Servant*

The *Diagnostic and Statistical Manual* (DSM-III, 1980) of the American Psychiatric Association (APA) and the World Health Organization's (WHO) *International Classification of Diseases* (ICD-9, 1977) list the following as mental disorders (DSM) or diseases (ICD): homosexuality; ego-dystonic homosexuality; fetishism; pedophilia; transvestism; exhibi-

---

Dr. Suppe is Professor of Philosophy, the Committee on the History and Philosophy of Science and Lecturer, School of Nursing at the University of Maryland. He is also consulting editor of the *Journal of Homosexuality*. This article draws from and incorporates portions of the author's chapters in the forthcoming, edited volume, *Medical Aspects of Human Sexuality* (ed. Earl Shelp). Partial support for this paper was provided by the University of Maryland General Research Board. Requests for reprints should be addressed to the author, Committee on the History and Philosophy of Science, 1131 Skinner Hall, University of Maryland, College Park, MD 20742.

tionism; voyeurism; sexual sadism; sexual masochism; zoophilia; transsexualism; gender identity disorder of childhood; various psychosexual dysfunctions such as inhibited sexual desire, excitement, and orgasm; and disorders of psychosexual identity, including feminism in boys.[1] Judged by current standards, these lists are curiously incomplete inasmuch as they exclude rape[2] and incest. These omissions are especially bewildering because DSM-III includes such unusual sexual disorders (under "Atypical Paraphilia," 320.90) as coprophilia, frotteurism, klismaphilia, mysophilia, necrophilia, telephone scatalogica, and urophilia (respectively, the eroticization of feces, rubbing, enemas, filth, corpses, obscene phone calling, and urination).

Prior to the Kinsey reports (Kinsey, Pomeroy, & Martin, 1948; Kinsey, Pomeroy, Martin, & Gebhard, 1953) there was a broad social consensus that the sexual practices catalogued in DSM and ICD were the marks of mentally ill persons. That consensus was destroyed by Kinsey's work, by later reports of the high incidence of homosexuality and bestiality, and by growing awareness of the variations in sexual practices.

The post-Kinsey sexual liberation has resulted in a wide variety of sexual practitioners stepping in with various sexual liberation movements, including the masochists (headquartered in the *Til Eulenspiegel* Society in New York), and the pederasts (e.g., the North American Man/Boy Love Association). The impetus of the Gay Liberation Movement also cannot be minimized. It not only has been a major influence in the decriminalization of homosexual behavior, but it has also played a major role in the removal of homosexuality *per se* from the DSM (Bayer, 1981; Suppe, 1982) and strengthens other segments of the sexual liberation movement.

The debates surrounding the declassification of homosexuality *per se* as a mental disorder in DSM-II, and their aftermath in the drafting of DSM-III (which includes ego-dystonic homosexuality but not homosexuality *per se*) raise questions not only about psychiatric evaluation of homosexuality, but also about sexual disorders in general. Specifically, the issue involves the extent to which such psychiatric evaluations are pseudo-scientific/medical masquerades of prevailing or reactionarily conservative social mores.

There is, in fact, good reason to suspect that the classifications of sexual paraphilias as mental disorders is the codification of social mores. The historical record clearly shows that in issues such as masturbation, abortion and contraception, venereal disease, and the inferiority of women and blacks, physicians have generally supported the prevailing mores, presenting research that gave credence and medico-scientific legitimacy to social prejudices (Bullough, 1963; Duffy, 1963, 1982; Englehardt, 1974; Haller & Haller, 1974). Lacking sufficient historical evidence to confirm this suspicion vis-à-vis homosexuality and the paraphilias, we will explore the issue by examining the APA decision to exclude homosexuality *per se* from DSM while adding ''ego-dystonic homosexuality,'' and then turn to a consideration of the inclusion of other sexual paraphilias as mental disorders.

EGO-DYSTONIC HOMOSEXUALITY AND THE CONCEPT OF A MENTAL DISORDER

As a result of lobbying that stressed research which challenged the prevailing psychiatric orthodoxy that homosexuality *per se* was an inevitable concomitant of psychopathology, the APA removed homosexuality *per se* from DSM-II in 1973. This decision was challenged by a group of psychiatrists headed by Irving Bieber and Charles Socarides, who forced a referendum vote of the APA membership. Gay activists attempted to defeat the referendum, and they succeeded: Homosexuality *per se* was no longer a mental disorder, although ''Sexual Orientation Disturbance'' (homosexuals who were ''disturbed by, in conflict with, or wish to change their sexual orientation'') was added to DSM-II. The episode was widely viewed as a breakdown of scientific objectivity in which politics and vested interests within and outside of psychiatry replaced reasoned debate and the canons of scientific evidence.

In 1974 the APA Task Force on Nomenclature and Statistics, led by Robert Spitzer (Note 1), was charged with preparing a new edition of DSM. The controversy over declassifying homosexuality prompted Spitzer and his committee carefully to examine and critically to rethink the very notion of a mental disorder.

This examination was clearly needed. Psychiatrists and philosophers have serious disagreements about the relationships among mental disorders, mental illness, and mental diseases. Some use the terms interchangeably while others attempt to draw sharp distinctions between them. DSM-III further complicates matters by including the category ''conditions not attributable to a Mental Disorder,'' which nevertheless are a focus of attention. Mental disorders also include short-term conditions such as alcohol intoxication, as opposed to alcoholism. The exact definition of ''mental disorder'' is increasingly unclear.

Spitzer and his committee were acutely aware of how problematic defining the concept of a mental disorder is, and went to considerable effort to try to produce a clear analysis of the concept. He wrote:

> When I first was given the job of considering the claims . . . that homosexuality should not be regarded as a mental disorder, I was confronted with the absence of any generally accepted definition of mental disorder. I therefore reviewed the characteristics of the various mental disorders and concluded that, with the exception of

homosexuality and perhaps some other "sexual deviations," they all generally cause subjective distress or were associated with generalized impairment in social effectiveness or functioning. It became clear to me that the *consequences* of a condition, and not its aetiology determined whether or not the condition should be considered a disorder. (Note 1, p. 5)

Although Spitzer eventually concluded that "no precise definition of disorder (physical or mental) was possible or even useful" (Note 1, p. 7), DSM-III does present "concepts" that have influenced decisions to include some conditions while excluding others. For example:

In DSM-III each of the mental disorders is conceptualized as a clinically significant behavioral or psychological syndrome or pattern that occurs in an individual and that is typically associated with either a painful symptom (distress) or impairment in one or more important areas of functioning (disability). In addition, there is an inference that there is a behavioral, psychological, or biological dysfunction, and that the disturbance is not only in the relationship between the individual and society. (When the disturbance is *limited* to a conflict between an individual and society, this may represent social deviance, which may or may not be commendable, but is not by itself a mental disorder. (Note 1, p. 6)

This statement does provide fairly explicit criteria for excluding homosexuality, left-handedness, and various forms of uncouth behavior from the list of mental disorders. But it obviously is not wholly adequate. Its employment, for instance, with regard to inclusion of the sexual paraphilias and ego-dystonic homosexuality is rather problematic. Before turning to such issues, some consequences of this statement need to be explored.

No precise definitions are given, as Spitzer noted, for key notions such as "impairment in one or more important areas of functioning" and "behavioral, psychologic, or biologic dysfunction" (Note 1, p. 8). He asserted that: "It should be understood that there is always a value judgment in deciding that a particular area of functioning is 'important'" (Note 1, p. 11). In short, when subjective distress is absent, whether a condition is a mental disorder is ultimately a value judgment and not a purely factual matter. Those such as Boorse (1975) who hold out for nonnormative conceptions of disease and illness surely will find this assertion wholly unacceptable. Also, given the extent to which clinical judgments of what is mentally healthy very strongly reflect sex-role stereotypes (Broverman, Broverman, Clarkson, Rosenkranz, & Vogel, 1970), Spitzer's definition of mental disorder would seem to license psychiatry to enforce social, political, and ideological conformity.

To be sure, Spitzer does not approve of psychiatric totalitarianism, and his definition of mental disorder does include specific caveats designed to block misapplications. However, the caveats seem futile. How does one distinguish impaired psychological functioning from "mere conflicts between an individual and society"? Spitzer seems to rely on consensus among psychiatrists and what he terms "the concept of inherent disadvantage" (Note 1, p. 11ff). Yet this idea does not come to grips with the issue. It would appear that, prior to Gay Liberation, when there was consensus that homosexuality *per se* was dysfunctional with inherent disadvantage, it *was* a mental disorder; now that the Gay Liberation Movement has raised doubts in so many therapists' minds and destroyed professional consensus, homosexuality no longer is a dysfunction, but is rather a conflict between society and the individual.

Does potential abuse of psychiatric diagnosis show that a normative, value-laden notion of mental disorder *ipso facto* is defective? No, because the notion of mental disorder, illness, or disease must be normative. Psychotherapeutic theories typically describe mechanisms whereby subsequent mental states are a function of earlier states. Some states are viewed as desirable (healthy) and others as undesirable (pathological). Because psychiatry is concerned with mental health, it has a normative set of mental states that exclude the pathological.

DSM-III's criteria for determining what are mental disorders, then, must be assessed on grounds of their normative adequacy. Precisely these issues were raised in the development of the manual in debates over the tenability of "Sexual Orientation Disturbances" as a mental disorder. Ultimately, the manual did include such a notion re-worded as "ego-dystonic homosexuality" (302.00), which has the following diagnostic criteria:

A. The individual complains that heterosexual arousal is persistently absent or weak and significantly interferes with initiating or maintaining wanted heterosexual relationships.
B. There is a sustained pattern of homosexual arousal that the individual explicitly states has been unwanted and a persistent source of distress. (p. 282)

Many experts (e.g., Paul Gebhard and John Money) argued against the inclusion of ego-dystonic homosexuality in DSM-III. They suggested that, if this were a legitimate category, it would be arbitrary to include it but exclude ego-dystonic heterosexuality, "distress over adulterous impulses," "ego-dystonic masturbation," and so on. Others thought it should be included under extant categories such as "Psychosexual Disorders not Elsewhere Classified" or various anxiety categories. Spitzer had a number of responses to this line of objection (Note 1, pp.

15–18), of which only the claim that there is no recorded instance of ego-dystonic heterosexuality in the literature was convincing.

Spitzer's responses do not address themselves to the more general problems concerning "ego-dystonic" categories. If ego-dystonic homosexuality, then why not also ego-dystonic psoriasis (better known as "the heartbreak of psoriasis"), ego-dystonic hemorrhoiditis (promoted by Preparation-H), ego-dystonic acnitis (promoted by Pat Boone, Clearasil, et al.), and ego-dystonic acomia (promoted by hair weaving, hair transplant, and wig firms)? In short, the range of symptoms that can be experienced by an individual as undesirable or alien—that is, ego-dystonic—boggles the imagination, and a decision to include homosexuality as the only ego-dystonic condition seems highly arbitrary and unwarranted. It raises the suspicion that the inclusion of ego-dystonic homosexuality is a codification of social mores.

This suspicion is reinforced by DSM-III's treatment of the so-called "sexual paraphilias," which are more in conflict with prevailing sexual mores than is homosexuality. The question arises whether the sexual paraphilias are any less a social deviance (limited to a conflict between an individual and society) than is homosexuality. If not, should the sexual paraphilias also be deleted from DSM? If deleted, would their replacement by ego-dystonic versions be justified?

SEXUAL PARAPHILIAS

One of the main groups of psychosexual disorders in DSM-III is the paraphilias. "The paraphilias are characterized by arousal in response to sexual objects or situations that are not part of *normative* arousal activity patterns and that in varying degrees *may interfere* with the capacity for reciprocal affectionate sexual activity" (p. 261, italics added). At the very heart of the DSM-III's thinking about the paraphilias is the idea that deviation from conventional sexual activity is unhealthy. The paraphilias listed in DSM-III are: Fetishism (302.81), Transvestism (302.30), Zoophilia (302.10), Pedophilia (302.20), Exhibitionism (302.40), Voyeurism (302.82), Sexual Masochism (302.83), Sexual Sadism (302.84), and Atypical Paraphilia (302.90), which is "a residual category for individuals with paraphilias that cannot be classified in any other categories."

The term "paraphilia" means "craving for the abnormal," but in sexology it has acquired the more specific meaning of requiring unusual objects, acts, or fantasies for sexual arousal and orgasm (Masters, Johnson, & Kolodny, 1982, pp. 342–343; Money, 1980, p. 220). DSM-III's characterization of paraphilia conforms with this standard usage:

[U]nusual or bizarre imagery or acts are necessary for sexual excitement. Such imagery or acts tend to be insistently and involuntarily repetitive and generally involve either (1) preference for use of a non-human object for sexual arousal, (2) repetitive sexual activity with humans involving real or simulated suffering or humiliation, or (3) repetitive sexual activity with nonconsenting partners. (p. 266)

But when DSM-III specifies diagnostic criteria for the paraphilias of fetishism, zoophilia, pedophilia, voyeurism, certain forms of sexual masochism, and sexual sadism, the requirements are loosened so that the use of such sources of excitement need only be a "repeatedly preferred or exclusive method of achieving sexual excitement" (p. 269; cf. pp. 270-273). With respect to transvestism, all that is required is "use of cross-dressing for the purposes of sexual excitement, *at least initially* in the course of the disorder" (p. 270, italics added). In the case of exhibitionism and certain forms of sexual sadism, *repetitive* occurrence of the acts is sufficient (pp. 272, 275). In certain forms of masochism and sadism, a single episode qualifies (pp. 274-275). Further, while DSM-III's definition of a paraphilia equates sexual activity and fantasy, the diagnostic categories for fetishism, exhibitionism, voyeurism, and sexual masochism require actual behavior. In most cases fantasy alone is explicitly disallowed from constituting a diagnosis. In the case of sexual sadism, the actions must be carried out or at least simulated. Only in zoophilia and pedophilia are overt activity and fantasy equated as the definition of paraphilia requires. Thus we see that the diagnostic requirements for specific paraphilias are often not consistent with DSM-III's own definition of a paraphilia.

Patterns of Sexual Response

An individual's *sexual identity* has the following distinct components: *biological sex* (whether one is male or female at birth); *gender identity* (one's basic conviction of being male or female); *social sex-role* (extent of conformity to physical and psychological characteristics culturally associated with males and females); and *sexual orientation,* which includes *sexual behavior* (patterns of erotic body contact with others), patterns of *interpersonal affection* (associations involving various degrees of trust such as with friends, lovers, and marital partners), *erotic fantasy structure* (sexually arousing patterns of mental images of one or more persons engaged in physical sexual activity or in affectional relationships), and *arousal cue-response patterns* (sensory cues which stimulate or inhibit erotic arousal) (Shively & DeCecco, 1977; Tripp, 1975; Note 2). Although sexual orientation is usually labeled bisexual, heterosexual, or homosexual, these labels can also be assigned to various components that may not be in accord with each other. Thus, one can be homosexual in some aspects of sexual orientation and heterosexual or bisexual in others.

It will be useful to expand our notions of sexual orientation to include more than just bisexuality, heterosexuality, and homosexuality. Sexual behavior can be expressed in the form of any of the paraphilias, as can fantasy structure or arousal cue-response patterns. With respect to various components of sexual orientation, an individual may be hetero-sexual, homosexual, bisexual, as well as fetishistic, transvestitic, zoophiliac, and so on. It is important to note that these are not mutually exclusive categories. For example, a female who is sexually aroused only by dressing in leather and being placed in bondage while fellating a male, with a dog performing cunnilingus, would be a heterosexual zoophiliac, fetishistic masochist.

By adolescence the individual has developed an idiosyncratic repertoire of highly specific cues that stimulate arousal. These may include, for ex-ample, various physiognomic features, circumstances, modes of dress, personality traits, modes of interpersonal behavior, smells, and music. Given the diversity of animate, inanimate, and situational cues that are routinely found in individual cue-response patterns, it is important to con-sider how these cues fit into the overall response pattern and to how domi-nant they are therein. The following classification is useful:

— *Inhibitory:* Cues that inhibit sexual arousal
— *Non-facilitative:* Cues that neither inhibit nor intensify sexual arousal
— *Facilitative:* Cues that enhance but are not necessary for sexual arousal
— *Paraphiliac:* Cues that are necessary for sexual arousal

Thus a person who was turned off by physical and psychological trauma would not be a masochist. But an individual whose sexual arousal was neither inhibited nor facilitated by such trauma would be a non-facilitative masochist. An individual who could get aroused without such trauma but found that spanking, hard bites, or verbal abuse increased arousal would be a facilitative masochist. An individual who, for in-stance, could only become aroused by having a stiletto heel ground into his testicles would qualify as a paraphiliac masochist. Similarly, we can talk of non-facilitative or facilitative forms of other paraphiliac acts.

Fairly close accord between sexual fantasies and arousal cue-response patterns is expected. While this frequently occurs (Masters et al., 1982, pp. 250–253), total accord between one's fantasy structure and arousal cue-response patterns is not always the case. Just as we can classify arousal cue-response patterns as homosexual, bisexual, heterosexual, fetishistic, masochistic, and so forth, so too can we classify erotic fantasy structures and distinguish between non-facilitative, facilitative, and paraphiliac fantasy ingredients.

Variant Sexual Disorders Reconsidered[3]

Recall that DSM-III allows activity or fantasy to qualify one for the diagnosis of zoophilia or pedophilia, but restricts fetishism, exhibitionism, voyeurism, and masochism to overt activity, and sadism to overt or simulated activity. Thus an individual who cannot be aroused except by fantasizing intercourse with a dog, but who is unwilling to do it in actuality, suffers from the mental disorder of zoophilia. On the other hand, an individual who cannot be aroused except by fantasies of being whipped as a sex slave in bondage, but who is unwilling to engage in such behavior, does not suffer a mental disorder. The difference here seems quite arbitrary.

Is there any rationale for including fantasy in zoophilia and pedophilia but not in the other paraphilias? The only clue I can find in DSM-III is that "the paraphilas . . . in varying degrees may interfere with the capacity for reciprocal affectionate sexual activity" (p. 261). In some cases, then, paraphiliac fantasy behavior would interfere with the capacity for reciprocal affectionate sexual activity and in others it would not. In discussing animal contacts, Kinsey, Pomeroy, and Martin (1948) write:

> In some cases the boy may develop an affectional relation with the particular animal with whom he has his contacts, and there are males who are quite upset emotionally when situations force them to sever connections with the particular animal . . . . The elements that are involved in sexual contacts between the human and animals of other species are at no point basically different from those that are involved in erotic responses to human situations . . . . On the other side of the record, it is to be noted that male dogs who have been masturbated may become considerably attached to the persons who provide the stimulation; and there are records of male dogs who completely forsake the females of their own species in preference for the sexual contacts that may be had with a human partner. (pp. 676–677)

It appears that in DSM-III it is the capacity for reciprocal affectionate activities with *adult humans* that makes the difference between pathological and nonpathological sexual behavior. If the paraphiliac fantasy structure is zoophiliac or pedophiliac, it will be problematic for an individual to respond sexually with adult humans. Although it might be difficult, it would not be impossible to copulate with an adult human while imagining a zoophiliac or pedophiliac episode. In such cases, the capacity for reciprocal affectionate activities with adult humans would exist, despite the paraphiliac fantasy structure. Acting out such fantasies is unlikely to be satisfying in the long term, however, and it is unlikely that such persons will be highly motivated to seek out adult human partners. Thus, in these cases, there does appear to be a rationale for including paraphiliac fantasy structures in the diagnoses of zoophilia and pedophilia.

Paraphiliac fantasy voyeurism and exhibitionism seem to have less potential for contributing to reciprocal affectionate activities with adult humans than do paraphiliac fantasy zoophilia or pedophilia. And the potential for paraphiliac fantasy fetishism is little better. For most of the variant sexual behaviors, then, the potential for paraphiliac fantasy interfering with the capacity for reciprocal affectionate activity with adult humans is similar in degree. Thus, my conclusion is that the decision to include fantasy in some, and exclude it in other, clinical diagnoses of paraphilias in DSM-III is arbitrary under the criterion of reciprocal affectionate activities.

The other side of the issue is whether paraphiliac arousal cue-response patterns fare any better on the reciprocal affection criterion. To the extent that exhibitionism or voyeurism requires the victims to be unsuspecting strangers, the opportunities for incorporating such paraphilias into reciprocal affectionate activities are even less for the paraphiliac fantasy forms. As noted above, the potential for reciprocal affection, with willing partners, is better in zoophilia or pedophilia. In fetishism, "reciprocal affection" depends largely upon the partner's comfort with, and ability to engage in, fetishistic activity.

The crucial cases thus become sexual sadism and masochism. Here we have the most complex interactions of paraphiliac fantasy and real life conditions, and also substantial potential for reciprocal affection. There are significant numbers of people whose sexual fantasies include masochism or sadism, with the former being in preponderance; but there are no reliable data as to what proportion, if any, is paraphiliac in fantasy structure. With respect to arousal cue-response, there appear to be significant numbers of people who are facilitative masochists, and somewhat fewer who are facilitative sadists. Whether there are any paraphiliac fantasy or arousal cue-response masochists or sadists is unclear because there are no reliable data on the subject. Nevertheless, S/M guides and books (e.g., Califia, 1980; Greene & Greene, 1974; Townsend, 1972) strongly suggest that: (1) the overwhelming majority of people involved in S/M activity are facilitative masochists; (2) much of S/M sex is psychodramatic acting out (simulation) among consensual partners, which minimizes actual physical or psychic trauma; (3) even facilitative sexual sadists are in the minority; (4) the shortage of participants who prefer the sexual sadist role is such that people preferring the sexual masochist role frequently, and often reciprocally, play the sadist role to keep the S/M psychodrama going. The picture gleaned from "insider" writings is that S/M typically involves high capacities for reciprocal affectionate sexual activities. Spengler (1979) confirms this portrait.

These observations, coupled with the paucity of empirical research on sexual sadism and masochism, and on the other "paraphilias," raises serious challenges. First, how many people actually meet the criteria for being paraphiliac with respect to fantasy structures or cue-response patterns for any of the DSM sexual variations? So far as I can tell from the literature and counseling contacts, they are extremely few. Rather, the norm is for quite a number to be facilitative in either fantasy or cue-response patterns with substantially more of the former. Second, the commercial success of S/M paraphernalia shops and interviews with their proprietors suggest that there are substantial numbers of couples who are capable of addressing their facilitative S/M fantasies and working them into consensual, cooperative, and affectionate sexual repertoire (my counseling experience reinforces this impression); and, in significant numbers of cases there is reason to believe that couples in which one member is a facilitative transvestite can do the same. Many couples break up over such fantasy structures and the expressed desire to act them out although there are substantial numbers who can incorporate them into productive, reciprocal, and affectionate relationships.

We conclude, then, that DSM-III offers no coherent rationale for its specific criteria for the inclusion and exclusion of specific patterns of variant sexual behavior.

Variant Sexual Behaviors as Psychological Disorders

Before it can be seen whether any justification exists for the continued inclusion of the "paraphilias" as mental disorders in DSM-III, we must first address a serious problem: the paucity and low quality of research on variant sexual behaviors. The situation is similar to that of research on homosexuality in the mid-sixties and earlier, in which a wealth of clinical data on mentally-disturbed homosexuals, some empirical research based on prison or psychiatric-patient samples, but very little research based on "normal" samples of homosexuals, existed. The portrait of homosexuality and its psychological correlates was greatly distorted, being based on highly biased samples. Subsequent research with non-clinical, non-prison samples radically changed our understanding of homosexuality, and was an important factor in the removal of homosexuality *per se* from DSM.

Research on other forms of variant sexual behavior catalogued in DSM-II includes an abundance of psychiatric case studies and theory. To a surprising degree, the theories show striking resemblance to the erroneous psychiatric theories that attempted to explain the inevitable psychopathology of homosexuality. For example, Charles Socarides' (1960) treatment of fetishism is based on pre-Oedipal identifications as is his account of homosexuality (1968). Virtually all the empirical studies are based on samples of arrested sex offenders; for only exhibitionism, transvestism, and pedophilia have substantial numbers of studies been done. For all the variations there is a paucity of research. In the area of sadomasochistic sex, the only empirical study based on a "normal" population is Spengler's (1979), which suggests that psychiatric views of S/M are as distorted as were earlier views of homosexuality.

These considerations suggest, but do not establish, that variant sexual behaviors *per se* should be removed from DSM, but that perhaps more restrictive versions (e.g., ego dystonias or disorders of impulse control) might legitimately be included.

The first question is whether paraphiliac instances of these disorders really exist (in fantasy or cue-response). We have no data that directly answer this question. Although "paraphilia" presently excludes homosexuality, given our use of "paraphiliac" and following DSM-II, we can talk of facilitative vs. paraphiliac homosexuality in fantasy and arousal. In a large study with the most representative homosexual sample yet, Bell and Weinberg (1978) found that 64% of the white homosexual males had engaged in heterosexual coitus; and that of those, 92% sometimes or always had reached orgasm (Table 3.4, pp. 286–288). Thus, the majority of their sample was not paraphiliac with respect to arousal cue response.[4] Twenty-three percent of the white male homosexuals had heterosexual masturbation fantasies. Thus, while the majority were apparently fantasy paraphiliac homosexuals, nearly a quarter were not. These data, coupled with the previously mentioned parallels between research on both homosexuality and the other variant behaviors, and my own sexual counseling experiences, strongly suggest to me that persons who are cue-response paraphiliac with respect to DSM-III's "paraphilias" are extremely rare, if they exist at all. I would, however, expect there to be substantially more individuals who are fantasy paraphiliacs.

Assuming that arousal cue-response paraphiliacs are so exceedingly rare, DSM-III's practice of not requiring the variant behaviors be paraphiliac, but rather only preferred, begins to make sense. Psychotherapists do encounter and attempt to treat people, e.g., for exhibitionism, fetishism, or pedophilia, either because a person is arrested for the behavior or because the behavior or fantasies are ego-dystonic; neither of these circumstances requires a paraphiliac response. In such cases the existence of a DSM classification for the paraphilias seems as appropriate as one for ego-dystonic homosexuality. The issue, of course, is whether DSM-III's current classifications are appropriate.

Recall that DSM-III conceptualizes mental disorders as significant behavioral or psychological syndromes typically associated with *distress* or *disability*. When the individual finds any of the variant sexual behaviors (or homosexuality or heterosexuality) ego-dystonic, then there is a case for including such behavior in DSM-III: It is the ego dystonia, not its sexual source, that warrants inclusion. The sexual ego dystonias, therefore, should be on an equal level with the non-sexual ones—perhaps in a generalized ego dystonia category. Whether such ego dystonias should be mental disorders (as opposed to being included among "Conditions not Attributable to a Mental Disorder that are a Focus of Attention or Treatment" is unclear for reasons discussed in Section I above.

Because many of the variant sexual behaviors (e.g., transvestism, sadism and masochism, fetishism) are often not ego-dystonic to the participants, under DSM-III's conceptualization the only grounds for including them *per se* as disorders would be if they inevitably lead to disability. Indeed, it was the conclusion that homosexuality *per se* did not inevitably lead to disability that contributed to its exclusion from DSM-III.

As discussed previously, DSM-III seems to view disability as an impairment of the capacity for reciprocal affectionate sexual activity between adult humans. A homosexual arousal cue-response pattern impairs the capacity for reciprocal affectionate sexual activity with adults of the opposite sex, but DSM-III judges that not to be a disability. But numerous male homosexuals choose to separate their affectionate behavior from their sexual activity, confining the latter to impersonal, non-affectionate, non-reciprocal activity. DSM-III evidently does not view such behavior as a disability, either. Instead, the judgment seems to be that homosexuals who reject reciprocal affectionate sexual activity are simply in conflict with society, rather than "disabled." DSM-III cannot view impaired capacity for reciprocal affectionate *sexual* activity as a disability in the case of the other variant behaviors while denying that it is for homosexuality. If the later merely constitutes a conflict between the individual and society, then *prima facie* so do the former.

The Specific "Disorders" Examined

Let us look more closely at one of the variant sexual behaviors in DSM-III, transvestism.[5] Some transvestites engage in ordinary coital behavior with their spouses and confine cross-dressing to solitary masturbation. Only if the wife becomes aware of the practice does it interfere with reciprocal affectionate behavior between them; in many cases the wife accepts the behavior and even cooperates in it (e.g., has sex with the husband while he is in drag). In other cases, however, the wife cannot accept it, and the relationship (sexual and affectionate) deteriorates. The situation here is not significantly different from that in which a heterosexually married person regularly engages in homosexual activity and is discovered by the spouse. Because, in the latter case, impairment of reciprocal affectionate activity does not qualify homosexuality *per se* to be included in DSM-III, by parity of reasoning neither should it qualify transvestism *per se*.

A larger issue here deserves treatment. Because one's arousal cue-re-sponse pattern is highly idiosyncratic, engaging in reciprocal affectionate sexual activity is effectively precluded with that part of the population that does not possess attributes complementary to one's cues. One has the ca-pacity to engage in sexual activity with a minority of people, and lacks it or has a limited capacity for it with respect to the majority. If transves-tism, homosexuality, or heterosexuality interferes with a relationship, one has picked the wrong partner. This can threaten the relationship, lead to unpleasant circumstances, and so forth, but it is not perforce a dis-order.

Similarly, not only do some individuals not eroticize affectionate or reciprocal sexual activity, but their arousal is inhibited by such activity. Their capacity for sexual activity is restricted to others who do not de-mand affection and reciprocity, or else find its absence erotic. In all these cases, variations in cue-response patterns may complicate partner selec-tion, but do not thereby constitute a disability. Rather, the situation is a conflict between an individual's arousal cue-response pattern and a socie-ty which says that sexual activity should be restricted to affectionate reciprocal activity without special props; this is so regardless of whether the socially disapproved cues are paraphiliac or facilitative.

Because "[f]etishes tend to be articles of clothing, such as female undergarments, shoes, and boots, or more rarely parts of the human body, such as hair or nails" (DSM-III, p. 268), fetishism is similar to transvestism, and the prior comments on capacity for reciprocal affec-tionate sexual activity apply *mutatis mutandis.* Even if the fetish is paraphiliac, which most are not, women do exist who find it arousing to wear heels and have men grovel at their feet licking their shoes; with such a partner the fetishist can work out a reciprocal affectionate psychodrama form of sexual activity.

Non-ego-dystonic fetishists typically receive treatment as a result of being arrested for stealing clothing (Masters et al., 1982, p. 343). Such compulsive behavior may qualify as a disability. On the other hand, not all behavior that is compulsive and illegal qualifies as a disability. The un-attached heterosexual who finds himself so sexually aroused that he haunts the singles bars to find a partner to fornicate with is engaging in compulsive behavior that in many jurisdictions is illegal (often a felony); yet we would tend to view this as fairly normal, not as a disability. Likewise, the fetishist who, on occasion, compulsively steals soiled pan-ties from baskets at the laundromat: the behavior is antisocial and a mis-demeanor, but it does not connote a serious disability. Only if the fetishist becomes so compulsively preoccupied with the fetish that he is seriously distracted from other responsibilities does it become a disability. This is the same as with any other form of sexual behavior. Thus, to the extent that fetishism is a disability, it is so by virtue of being a "Disorder of Impulse Control" and should be so classified, just as ego-dystonic fetishism should be classified with other non-sexual ego dystonias.

With regard to sadomasochism, DSM-III focuses on sadism and masochism as involving suffering, and being dangerous to life or limb. In the case of sexual sadism, but not of sexual masochism, psychodrama ("simulation") or mild physical trauma qualifies for inclusion. When confined to episodes that are psychodramatic in nature or involve trauma whose effects do not interfere with other activities more than, say, equally unanticipated sports-related injuries, it is difficult to see how participation in S/M constitutes a disability. Moreover, with suitably matched partners, sadomasochistic activities can be genuinely reciprocal and affectionate.

What about the sexual masochist, of which there are at best few, who wants and allows himself to be maimed, harmed, or killed? Clearly, a disability exists, and some sort of mental disorder is present. It may help if we compare Asphyxiophilia (repetitive erotic hangings). It is well known that when males are executed by hanging they frequently get erections and ejaculate. Burroughs (1959) has glorified this in a passage ("Hassan's Rumpus Room," pp. 74–83). Some individuals attempt to obtain this thrill, without dying, by having a partner cut them down before death occurs. The closest applicable criterion in DSM-III would be: "The individual has intentionally participated in activity in which he or she was physically harmed or his or her life was threatened, in order to produce sexual excitement" (p. 274).

An individual I interviewed had intentionally participated in these hangings on three occasions, but was not harmed. He had no desire to die or expectation that he would, he felt that the risk of serious harm or death was minimal, and his partner was skilled in the activity. While there was a small chance of death, it is not clear that his life was threatened. At the same time, I can see how others might reasonably insist that he intentionally risked or threatened his life.

Nevertheless, the case is quite different from suicide or death- or mutilation-wish behavior. Whereas we plausibly would view the latter as evidence of a mental disorder (though it is not so classified in DSM), we do not generally brand daredevils who know what they are doing as mentally disordered just because they take serious risks. It seems to me that masochistic activity takes on the form of a disability either when it becomes a compulsive behavior that seriously interferes with other responsibilities, or else when it has as its focus being maimed, crippled, or killed. In such cases the disability, hence the disorder, seems only incidentally sexual, and participants would better be classified under some other personality or dysthemic (depressive) disorder.

Similarly, the sexual sadist who goes beyond the consensual psycho-drama (i.e., the agreed-upon levels of non-maiming trauma), and inflicts excessive, permanent, or mortal injury on a sexual partner seems more appropriately classified under "Antisocial Personality Disorder" (301.70) or "Adult Antisocial Behavior" (V71.01; see also p. 319).

Exhibitionistic behavior tends to be highly compulsive and includes uncontrollable urges; it typically involves an unsuspecting victim. DSM-III's diagnostic criteria for it are "repetitive acts of exposing the genitals to an unsuspecting stranger *for the purpose of achieving sexual excitement,* with no attempt at further sexual activity with the stranger" (p. 272; italics added).

This classification is rather problematic because not all exhibitionists are able to achieve an erection or to ejaculate during the exposure episode (Lester, 1975; Masters et al., 1982, p. 347); it is unclear whether, or how, sexual exhibitionism is, in fact, rooted in the arousal cue-response patterns of the individual. This suggests that it would be more appropriately classified under the "Antisocial Personality Disorder," "Adult Antisocial Behavior," or "Disorders of Impulse Control" categories.

Voyeurism may or may not be ego-dystonic. To the extent it is a disability, it is one because non-consenting persons are viewed; this minimizes the ways of incorporating it productively into interpersonal sexual activity that do not run afoul of the law, but does not preclude the possibility. The danger of arrest does not make voyeurism any more a mental disorder than does the illegality of homosexual acts in many jurisdictions. To the extent that voyeurism warrants classification in DSM, it should fall under the various antisocial or impulse disorders already mentioned.

Zoophilia has been discussed previously. To the extent that an individual—even if arousal-cue paraphiliac—can participate in reciprocal and affectionate sexual behavior with animals and can otherwise participate normally in society, there seems no disability worthy of inclusion *per se* in DSM. Zoophilia may or may not be ego-dystonic.

I turn now to the most controversial form of variant behavior in DSM—pedophilia. DSM-III restricts pedophilia to sex between adults and pre-pubescent children. This means that it excludes sex between adults and pubescent children who do not have fully developed genitals and who are incapable of ovulating or ejaculating, as well as between adults and early adolescents.[6] Many would find DSM-III's classification unduly narrow by virtue of excluding contact with pubescents and early adolescents and would disagree that "[i]solated sexual acts with children do not warrant the diagnosis of Pedophilia" (p. 271), and would further reject the idea that the acts must be "a repeatedly preferred or exclusive method of achieving sexual excitement" (p. 272) in order to qualify them as a sexual disorder.

The extent to which pedophilia is ego-dystonic to either the adult or the child is unclear. However, "[t]he child . . . is rarely as totally ingenuous or helpless as in the stereotype; the older the child, the more likely he is to have consented or even participated actively" (Detre & Jarecki, 1971, p. 272).[7]

Much of pedophiliac behavior is incestuous. Although the research literature is considerably biased to the effect that incest is the behavior of psychologically disturbed individuals, evidence exists to suggest that incestuous behavior can occur without any psychological harm to the participants, and that when harm does occur it is sometimes due primarily to the trial and incarceration of the parent. Indeed, it has been hypothesized that there is greater potential for psychological harm to post-adolescent children than to preadolescent ones (Lester, 1975, ch. 15, esp. pp. 131, 141). All of this suggests that at least some pedophiliac experiences are not ego-dystonic for adult or child; however, this is not intended to minimize the fact that there are many traumatic pedophiliac and incestuous occurrences.

Does pedophilia inevitably result in disability? Data on the subject are scarce, and most are based on arrested sex offenders. The best available data concerns homosexual pederasts involved with adolescent boys. Tindall (1978) followed, for up to 30 years, a large group of male adolescents involved for some duration with older men. His results were surprising: The youths all turned out to be well-adjusted, heterosexual adults who retrospectively felt the pederastic relationship has been most valuable. Typically, at the time of the pederastic involvement, the youths had been troublemakers who needed ongoing involvement with, and the support and understanding of, sympathetic adults. They did not receive such support at home, but found it in the pederastic relationship and productively exploited it to their own benefit.

My own interviews with pederasts tend to bear this out. They report that their primary concern is parenting a youth who needs support and is not getting it at home; while they desire sexual contact with the adolescents, they do not demand it. Surprisingly, they report that the youth's parents often know about and approve of the relationships. This strongly suggests that pedophilia with pubescents and post-pubescents need not constitute a disability for the youth or the adult.[8]

This tells us little about pre-pubescent or heterosexual pedophilia; reliable data are rare on these subjects. Money (1980) does claim that matching of a pedophiliac with a partner who provides genuine erotic reciprocity "is more common than conventionally believed" (p. 84). Pre-adolescent pedophilia typically involves not strangers, but relatives or others well-known to the child (Detre & Jarecki, 1971; Lester, 1975); pedophilia tends to be less psychologically damaging to pre-adolescents than to post-adolescents. These facts, together with what is known about post-adolescent pedophilia, suggest that the potential exists for some pre-pubescent pedophiliac relationships to be rewarding to both participants in ways analogous to the adolescent cases.

On the other hand, in those cases in which pedophiliac involvement is not consensual and reciprocal, where coercion is involved, and where the nurturing "parental" role is missing, real potential exists for psychological damage to the child. In such cases, however, the most appropriate DSM classification would be under the "Antisocial Behavior," "Personality Disorders," or "Disorders of Impulse Control" classifications already mentioned.

The foregoing considerations are, admittedly, somewhat speculative, although they are based on the limited evidence available. To the extent they are sound, they strongly suggest that, under DSM-III's concept of a mental disorder, pedophilia *per se* should not be automatically included in DSM.

CONCLUSIONS

My discussion of variant sexual behaviors exploits the limited available empirical research evidence to suggest that none of the variant behaviors *per se*, even if arousal cue-response paraphiliac (and even less so if fantasy paraphiliac), automatically warrants inclusion in DSM as a mental disorder. In effect, the same sorts of considerations that prompted the removal of homosexuality *per se* and the attendant rethinking of the criteria for a mental disorder in DSM-III, if consistently applied, also call for the removal of the other variant sexual behaviors.

To be sure, the available research data are uneven, sparse, and unreliable. But the data that support the inclusion of such disorders are even sparser and weaker. In the absence of reliable data based upon non-clinical, non-criminal samples in well-designed and executed studies, it is irresponsible to include such variations *per se* or even their paraphiliac versions in DSM-III. I have tried to show that the best available evidence provides a plausible basis for excluding the paraphilias *per se* from DSM. Manifestations of such behaviors warrant inclusion only when ego dystonias associated with them are on an equal level with non-sexual ego dystonias, or else when they fall into other antisocial behavioral, personality[9] or impulse control disorder categories.

This investigation of the so-called "sexual paraphilias" in DSM has reinforced the suspicion that they are not, *per se,* mental disorders, but rather constitute conflicts between an individual and society. Their inclusion in DSM-III is unwarranted, unscientific, and only serves to strengthen the conclusion that psychiatry has resorted to the codification of social mores while masquerading as an objective science. Indeed, even if this suspicion is incorrect, the burden of proof rests with psychiatry.

NOTES

1. In a few cases (e.g., ego-dystonic homosexuality vs. homosexuality or differences in nomenclature) the diagnostic classifications are not in total agreement.

2. Feminist writings on the subject argue that rape is an act of violence, not of sexuality. In support, it appears to be the case that there is a high incidence of impotence on the part of rapists (Groth & Burgess, 1977). Whether rape is a sexual disorder or not, it ought to appear in DSM-III. Similar comments apply to incest, at least that which is coercive.

3. Because I have adopted the term "paraphiliac" as part of my classification scheme, I will, for the most part, refer to the behaviors DSM calls paraphilias as *variant sexual behaviors.*

4. Their sample of homosexuals included people who were bisexual in behavior; nevertheless, 74% of the white males were currently exclusively homosexual in their behavior. For simplicity, I am reporting only data from white males here; the figures are higher for black homosexual males and for females.

5. For surveys of the literature on variant sexual behaviors that substantiate various claims made in the following discussion, see Lester (1975) and Masters et al. (1982, Ch. 14).

6. Much of the literature construes pedophilia to include sex between adults and pre-pubertal, pubertal, and early-adolescent individuals. Puberty may take six months to six years to complete. The ability to ovulate or ejaculate occurs late in puberty.

7. Detre and Jarecki (1971, p. 272) base the claim on *California Sexual Deviation Research: Preliminary Report,* January 1953, State of California, Department of Mental Hygiene, The Langley-Porter Clinic, Sacramento; and their Final Report, March 1954.

8. A fascinating novel about homosexual pederasty that displays these attitudes and perspectives is Dukahz (1966). The reports in Rossman (1976) tend to confirm this portrait.

9. Challenges to the legitimate classification of antisocial or personality disorders as mental disorders—as opposed to conflicts between an individual and society—are beyond the scope of this essay, as are considerations of the viability of DSM-III's concept of what constitutes a mental disorder.

REFERENCE NOTES

1. Spitzer, R. (1980). Homosexuality and mental disorder: A reformulation of the issues. Working paper, Hastings Center Closure Project.

2. Suppe, F. Changing sexual orientation: The moral issues, forthcoming in R. Baker and F. Elliston (Eds.), *Philosophy and sex* (2nd ed.). Buffalo: Prometheus Books.

REFERENCES

American Psychiatric Association. (1968). *Diagnostic and statistical manual of mental disorders* (2nd ed.). Washington, DC.

American Psychiatric Association. (1980). *Diagnostic and statistical manual of mental disorders* (3rd ed.). Washington, DC.

Bayer, R. (1981). *Homosexuality and American psychiatry.* New York: Basic Books.

Bell, A., & Weinberg, M. (1978). *Homosexuality: A study of diversity among men and women.* New York: Simon and Schuster.

Boorse, C. (1975). On the distinction between disease and illness. *Philosophy and Public Affairs, 5,* 49–68.

Broverman, I., Broverman, D. M., Clarkson, F. E., Rosenkranz, P. S., & Vogel, S. R. (1970). Sexrole stereotypes and clinical judgments of mental health. *Journal of Consulting and Clinical Psychology, 34,* 1–7.

Bullough, V. L. (1976). *Sexual variance in society and history.* Chicago: University of Chicago Press.

Burroughs, W. (1959). *Naked lunch.* New York: Grove Press.

Califia, P. (1980). *Sapphistry: The book of lesbian sexuality.* Tallahassee: Naiad Press.

Coleman, E. (1982). Developmental stages in the coming-out process. In W. Paul, J. D. Weinrich, J. C. Gonsiorek, & M. E. Hotvedt (Eds.), *Homosexuality: Social, psychological, and biological issues.* Beverly Hills, CA: Sage Publications.

Detre, T. P., & Jarecki, H. (1971). *Modern psychiatric treatment.* Philadelphia: Lippincott.

Duffy, J. (1963). Masturbation and cliteridectomy. *Journal of the American Medical Association, 186,* 246-248.

Duffy, J. (1982). The physician as a moral force in American history, In W. B. Bondeson, H. T. Englehardt, Jr., S. F. Spicker, & J. M. White, Jr. (Eds.), *New knowledge in the biomedical sciences.* Dordrecht: Reidel.

Dukahz, C. (1966). *The asbestos diary.* New York: Oliver Layton Press.

Englehardt, H. T., Jr. (1974). The disease of masturbation: Values and concepts of disease. *Bulletin of the History of Medicine, 47,* 234-238.

Englehardt, H. T., Jr., (1977). Is there a philosophy of medicine? In F. Suppe & P. Asquith (Eds.), *PSA 1976, 2.* East Lansing, MI: Philosophy of Science Association.

Greene, G., & Greene, C. (1974). *S-M — The last taboo: A study of sadomasochism.* New York: Grove Press.

Groth, A. M., & Burgess, A. W. (1977). Sexual destruction during rape. *New England Journal of Medicine, 297,* 764-766.

Haller, J. S., Jr., & Haller, R. M. (1974). *The physician and sexuality in victorian America.* Urbana: University of Illinois Press.

Kinsey, A., Pomeroy, W., & Martin, C. (1948). *Sexual behavior in the human male.* Philadelphia: W. B. Saunders.

Kinsey, A., Pomeroy, W., Martin, C., & Gebhard, P. (1953). *Sexual behavior in the human female.* Philadelphia: W. B. Saunders.

Lester, D. (1975). *Unusual sexual behavior: The standard deviations.* Springfield, IL: Charles C. Thomas.

Masters, W. H., Johnson, V. E., & Kolodny, R. C. (1982). *Human sexuality.* Boston: Little Brown.

Money, J. (1980). *Love and love sickness: The science of sex, gender difference, and pair-bonding.* Baltimore: John Hopkins University Press.

Rossman, P. (1976). *Sexual experience between men and boys.* New York: Association Press.

Socarides, C. (1960). The development of a fetishistic perversion. *Journal of the American Psychoanalytic Association, 8,* 281-311.

Socarides, C. (1968). *The overt homosexual.* New York: Grune & Stratton.

Shively, M., & DeCecco, J. (1977). Components of sexual identity. *Journal of Homosexuality, 3,* 41-48.

Spengler, A. (1979). *Sadomasochisten und ihre Subkulturen.* Frankfurt/Main: Campus Verlag.

Suppe, F. (1982). Review of R. Bayer, *Homosexuality and American psychiatry. Journal of Medicine and Philosophy, 7,* 375-381.

Tindall, R. H. (1978). The male adolescent involved with a pederast becomes an adult. *Journal of Homosexuality, 1978, 3,* 373-382.

Townsend, L. (1972). *The leatherman's handbook.* San Francisco: LeSalon.

Tripp, C. A. (1975). *The homosexual matrix.* New York: McGraw-Hill.

World Health Organization. (1977). *Manual of the international statistical classification of diseases, injuries, and causes of death.* 9th rev., 2 vols. Geneva: Author.

The Ethical and Moral Implications of Sexual Classification: A Commentary

Charles Silverstein, PhD
New York City

ABSTRACT. This paper reviews the relationship between psychiatric diagnosis and morality, suggesting that moral reasoning has been the primary determinant in the diagnosis of sexual disorders. It suggests two hypotheses to explain why homosexuality was eliminated from DSM. One, that homosexuality is now viable as a lifestyle and therefore has become socially regulated; and two, that the normal is the intractible. It further suggests that there is no scientific reason to keep the paraphilias in DSM.

A close relationship has always existed between moral beliefs and medical, particularly psychiatric, diagnosis and treatment. Historians have described how ancient and medieval beliefs influenced the diagnosis and treatment of the insane (Foucault, 1973; Rosen, 1968; Szasz, 1970). Halleck (1971), in addition, noted the political implications of medical diagnosis in present-day practice.

Many of the most renowned historical figures in psychiatry demonstrate the degree to which their professional beliefs were molded by the morality of their times. In France, for instance, Pinel, famous for removing the chains from the patients at Bicêtre and Salpetrière in 1794, stressed the benefits of moral treatment, including kindness, careful coercion and work therapy. Foucault (1973) views Pinel's treatment as a technique for socializing people to the values of a bourgeois society, including obedience, work and property values.

Dr. Silverstein is licensed as a psychologist in the states of New York and New Jersey. He was the founding editor of the *Journal of Homosexuality*. He is the author of several books, including *The Joy of Gay Sex* (with Edmund White) and *Man to Man: Gay Couples in America*. He is currently conducting an in-depth survey of the masturbatory fantasies of men and women. A version of this paper was presented at the 16th annual convention of the Association for the Advancement of Behavior Therapy, Los Angeles, 19-21 November, 1982. Requests for reprints should be addressed to the author, 233 West 83rd Street, New York, NY 10024.

At about the same time in the young American republic, Benjamin Rush led the development of psychiatry and diagnosed a variety of behaviors as medical problems, including lying, drunkenness and crime (Conrad & Schneider, 1980).[1] A fierce advocate of independence from England and a signer of the Declaration of Independence, Rush diagnosed anyone opposing the revolution as suffering from the disease of "revolutiona." He was an early and active abolitionist, basing his convictions partly on the belief that blacks had a disease called "negritude," which was inherited from ancestors with leprosy and which had turned their skins black (Conrad & Schneider, 1980).

While Rush may have been the medical advocate for abolition, Samuel Cartwright, a southern physician, represented the slavery side of the argument. In 1851, Cartwright published a paper describing the disease "drapetomania," a condition that only affected slaves, "and whose major symptom was running away from the plantation of their white masters" (Conrad & Schneider, 1980, p. 35).

Finally, mid-nineteenth-century feminists, in contrast to feminists of today, opposed abortion as dangerous to women's health and symptomatic of the oppression of women. The feminists allied themselves with the newly organized American Medical Association and lobbied state legislatures to outlaw abortion before "quickening" (fetal movement).[2] Physicians who were members of the new American Medical Association were struggling for medical primacy over other medical and non-medical groups, and saw in the anti-abortion statutes a means of creating a medical monopoly. The legislators—native-born, white Americans—were finding that middle- and upper-class women were having abortions, while waves of lower class immigrants with large families were arriving in America, and they felt betrayed by their own women. What they wanted was more native, Protestant babies to save America from the foreigners (Mohr, 1978). Beginning with post-Civil War America, women who desired abortion (or contraceptives, or who masturbated) were sometimes subjected to clitoridectomies and castration (Barker-Benfield, 1975).

Since the end of World War II, and most notably with the rise of the Gay Liberation movement, a controversy has arisen concerning what opinion mental health practitioners should take regarding the mental status of homosexuality. Some practitioners (Begelman, 1977; Davison, 1977; Silverstein, 1977) argue that moral reasoning alone contributes to defining homosexuality as a mental disorder, and they maintain that it is immoral to attempt sexual reorientation. Less radical are the positions of Marmor (1965), Green (1972), and Bell and Weinberg (1978), who also believe that homosexuality should no longer be considered a mental illness, but who do not consider sexual reorientation immoral for those men and women who find a homosexual life an alien one.

Opposed, for the most part, are the psychoanalysts (e.g., Bieber, Dain,

Dince, Drellich, Grand, Gundlach, Kremer, Rifkin, Wilber, and Bieber, 1962; Hatterer, 1970; Socarides, 1975), but also a number of behaviorists (e.g., Bancroft, 1974; Feldman, 1977), who not only believe that homosexuality is a psychological disturbance of the worst sort (the psychoanalytic view), but also that it is immoral to withhold treatment from those members of society who find their homosexuality painful and, therefore, wish to be reoriented.

These two groups have been at loggerheads, debating both the moral and therapeutic considerations of sexual reorientation, and in 1972 they lobbied the American Psychiatric Association's Committee on Nomenclature for either the retention or deletion of homosexuality as a mental disorder. Through a series of both professional discussions and political negotiating, the American Psychiatric Association removed homosexuality *per se* as a mental disorder in 1973 (APA, Note 1). In 1975, the American Psychological Association went on record as supporting the change.

The strategies and undercurrents of this change are reported from a positive viewpoint in Conrad and Schneider (1980), and critically by Socarides (1975). By far the most carefully researched book on the negotiations that led up to the change is Bayer (1981). While the moves and parries of the various parties to this controversy have been amply discussed in print, one is still left wondering why the membership of the American Psychiatric Association voted to remove homosexuality *per se* as a disorder, an action that is still seen as controversial. This is particularly intriguing, because a survey by *Medical Aspects of Human Sexuality* (1977) found that most psychiatrists still believe that homosexuality is not normal. Most interesting to ponder for those interested in sex research is the extent to which the current diagnostic system is still contaminated by diagnoses included for moral reasons, with little or no foundation in scientific judgment.

Why was homosexuality removed as a disorder in 1973? The psychiatrists said it was because the psychological research placed before them (e.g., Silverstein, 1976/1977; Wilson, Note 2) demonstrated that homosexual men and women were indistinguishable from heterosexuals. However, such changes do not usually occur because of advances in knowledge. Two alternate explanations suggest themselves. The first is that homosexuality no longer seems so abnormal because it is increasingly common, not in the sense of there being more homosexuals, but in that it is more feasible to live one's life as a homosexual in today's society.

Homosexuality has lost its status as a secret. It is no longer a plant kept in a dark closet that blooms only when brought into the well-lit office of the psychologist or psychiatrist. One might almost say that it was the circumstances in which information was divulged that rendered it abnormal or normal. What was sin?—that which was divulged in the confessional.

What was abnormal?—that which was divulged in the professional office.

Perhaps the sex crimes with social credentials, e.g., rape, incest, or adultery, are not on the official list because they are, and have been, public too long. It is preeminently the secret and the solitary, what people have kept to themselves out of pride or fear, private property par excellence, that have been listed in the DSM. Whether society truly abhors these acts as acts or whether it resents their being excluded from its supervision and control is another question. Perhaps the abnormal is merely the socially unregulated.

Another explanation may be attempted. Desire has a long history. The Greeks said that it preceded mankind itself. Christianity, with a much shorter history, cast a baleful eye at this competitor with a longer pedigree, and pronounced it sinful. The avowed aim of the church was to extirpate desire, but she wisely contented herself with suppressing it, with making it into a secret. Let desire go with a black veil over its face, and silently, too. This is the genesis of the least naive of the virtues, chastity.

We, moderns, are more sympathetic than the Christians. Desire can walk the streets once more and even hold its head up, but only, for we are still living in a Judeo-Christian society, when it goes hand in hand with an appropriate object and has an appropriate aim in mind.[3] This is the hubris of modern psychological and psychiatric treatment. We are not content to smother homosexual desire, to make sure that that love never even whispers its name, but courageously dream of correcting it, directing it, and reorganizing it from homosexual to heterosexual.

But sexuality resists psychological theories, particularly those based upon a foundation of morality rather than empiricism. None of the attempts to change homosexuals into heterosexuals has met with any lasting success, the claims of psychoanalysts (Bieber et al., 1962) and some behavior therapists (Feldman & MacCulloch, 1971) notwithstanding.

Perhap chagrin at this failure contributed to the readiness with which homosexuality was removed from DSM. The uncomfortable thought one is left with is the equation of the normal with the intractable. Maybe homosexuality is no longer judged abnormal because many professionals feel they can do nothing to change it.

Now let us assume that we are all determinists, and that we all believe that if we could chart all of the variables of a person's life we would completely understand why one person acts differently from another and how and why one person changes over time. Let us further assume that we would find variations in the psychological and cultural backgrounds, and that these differences might explain the variations in people's behavior. But by what criteria do we differentiate between a behavioral variation and a pathological act? The distinction was very clear before DSM-III (1980); that which was judged immoral was invariably also illegal and, hence, pathological. The removal of homosexuality has now opened the question of whether the same arguments used to justify this action may be applied to other sexual disorders.

The paraphilias in DSM-III (1980) are essentially the same as in DSM-II (1968), where they were called sexual deviations. They have at least two things in common: They appear "kinky" to us and none of them leads to coitus and reproduction. They are, in the words of St. Thomas Aquinas, all *contra naturam,* against nature. We should note the absence of two other sexual behaviors from all the DSMs—rape and incest—that are predominantly heterosexual, frequently involve coitus and can lead to reproduction. There is no reason to believe that a man who coerces his young daughter into sexual acts is any less worthy of an honored place on the list than someone who peeps through his neighbor's window at night.

What am I to think of a patient of mine, a confirmed masochist, who experiences love and fulfillment while being humiliated? Or another patient who, in addition to "vanilla sex" with his lover, participates in scatological scenes with strangers? What am I to think of a third patient whose masturbatory fantasies have him taking care of and having sex with a young boy?

Res ipsa loquitur is a legal expression that means the thing speaks for itself. The professional community has implicitly agreed that the acts of these patients speak for themselves, and they they are offensive, abnormal, and therefore appropriate for behavioral change. But if we are to maintain our intellectual integrity, perhaps we ought to use the removal of homosexuality as an opportunity to redefine sexual behavior by empirical means rather than by relying on Judeo-Christian morality. *Res ipsa loquitur* is not a psychological term, nor is *contra naturum.* We do not have the knowledge today to distinguish between a behavioral variation and an abnormality, and we should no longer pretend that we do.

It is my belief that combining moral beliefs and psychological judgments shows a lack of respect for both; that it minimizes the importance of moral standards in society as well as the potential contributions of psychology. Popper (1959) correctly maintained that no amount of scientific evidence can prove or disprove a moral belief. Moral beliefs are independent of psychological processes. For instance, many of us believe that a rapist should be sent to jail for a very long time. Suppose this rapist is found to have had a miserable home life, an abusive father, a drunken mother (whose pregnancy was deficient in the proper nutrients), and terrible teachers in a ghetto school. In short, he learned very bad habits. Would we excuse his behavior because, as determinists, we maintain that the cause of the rape was improper schedules of reinforcement, or a faulty resolution of the Oedipus complex, and absolve him of responsibility? The law, the enforcing arm of morality, says "Put him in jail," regardless of the results of an MMPI or a Rorschach. Our legal code requires that the rest of us should be protected from a rapist regardless of the motivation for the rape. From the standpoint of psychology, rape is neither good nor bad behavior, but merely the endpoint of a series of variables that psychology can, and probably should, examine.

As members of society we have every right to be outraged by a person's immoral behavior without seeking to point to some abnormality as the cause. I felt that way when I read the Holyroyd and Brodsky (1977) study on sexual contact between psychologists and their patients. We should be able to demonstrate that a person's sexual behavior is abnormal, even though it does not violate moral beliefs. A man who refuses to have sex with his wife because of his delusion that she is the Virgin Mary may be such an example.

But now what of the middle-aged man who prefers to have consensual sex with his wife by watching her masturbate while he's dressed in women's lingerie, wearing a Bella Abzug-like hat? What of the women who prefers to act out her rape fantasies with her trusted lover who pretends to take her by force while she pretends to resist him? And what of a gay man with an appetite for sexual novelty so great that he can count thousands of sexual partners in his lifetime? These are all adult sexual behaviors with adult consenting partners, in private, that bring sexual pleasure to the participants. Yet each would be judged immoral, if not outright weird, by most Americans. They are indeed atypical behaviors, at least by statistical standards, but where is the evidence, beyond *res ipsa loquitur,* that they are abnormal or inappropriate? If, as we did with homosexuality, we compared test results between people who indulge in the paraphilias and the rest of us, and found no difference, wouldn't we have to insist that they be removed from DSM? The answer could only be "Yes."

The removal of homosexuality as a DSM disorder was a magnificent political move meant to assimilate gay people into the majority, and hence more them towards the standards of the heterosexual world. I think it was a stroke of genius on the part of those psychiatrists who were insightful enough to see that being homosexual was no longer a secret, was immune to treatment, and that labeling homosexuality abnormal caused unnecessary suffering in otherwise productive people. And they could effect this revolution without a significant change in the moral foundation of the sexual disorders category in DSM. Happy gays, no longer abnormal, would form relationships based largely on a copy of heterosexual marriage. Apart from the happy homosexuals are the real deviants, people suffering from gender identity problems, the paraphiliacs, and unhappy homosexual men and women.

The distinction between happy homosexuality and the paraphilias is arbitrary. We have no concrete evidence that the paraphilias are any more or less normal or abnormal than homosexuality, and we are pleased to allow them to remain in DSM because they offend us. If we had more integrity we would insist that either empirical evidence of their abnormality be produced or that they be dropped from DSM. Only Money (1977, 1981) has written extensively on the paraphilias with the intent of gaining scientific knowledge about them as part of a comprehensive understanding of human sexuality.

Our current models of sexual behavior are poorly constructed. The moral (Sedgwick, 1973) is based upon how we insist people should behave, rather than what behaviors they prefer. There is then Freud's libido model, a hydraulic system so comprehensive that it tells us everything about all levels of behavior, hence nothing at all about sexuality. Behavior theory tells us very little about sexuality *per se,* assuming that the same laws for learning cognitive functions also rule sexuality. In my opinion, the best theory of sexuality (or, at least, male sexuality) is a Yiddish proverb that says, "When the penis is hard, the brains are soft."

A bit mischievously, I can suggest two standards for moral behavior. We might propose, for example, a model of sexuality where abnormality is defined by the predictability and limitations of the sexual behavior of the participants. As we all know, boredom—not lack of desire—is the greatest sexual problem in long-lasting relationships, heterosexual and homosexual. Normality might be defined as unpredictability, creativity, and spontaneity in the participants and how fresh and alive they feel when they arise in the morning. Old sexual standbys would be integrated with role reversals, kinky paraphilias, sexual toys, and whatever other ideas occurred to the participants to increase or decrease sexual excitement as they desired.

Playing with this idea of alternate models, we might propose that having a sexual identity is abnormal, and not having one is normal. The historically minded psychologist will surely note that history would be on our side, because the term "homosexual" was only coined in 1869, and "heterosexual" became a sexual identity only a few decades later.

An an aside, I would also like to note that the list of sexual disorders is almost completely a list of male behaviors. I am always amazed that so few clinicians and researchers take note of this. Harmful, or merely atypical, men probably make up at least 90% of those diagnosed. One might reasonably remark that the virtual monopoly of men diagnosed as the sexually bizarre is an evolutionary quirk. Ignoring that the sexual disorder list is a male list is to refuse to consider what implications the fact has for any model of sexuality.

I do not know if it is possible to rid psychology of its moral background, or whether that is even desirable. Nor do I believe that psychologists should be morally neutral in their own beliefs. I am not prepared to tell a psychologist how to deal with a patient who desperately begs him or her to remove a sexual behavior the psychologist might judge as psychologically harmless, nor am I prepared to condemn as fascist any psychologist who would treat such a person. I would, however, ask why he or she is doing so. At the moment I want only to begin thinking about sexuality in new ways and to try to make decisions about what to carry on from the past, and this means distinguishing between historical wisdom and dead wood.

Around the middle of the eighteenth century, a Swiss physician named Tissot wanted to find a physiological basis for morality. He found it in the putative harmfulness of masturbation, which caused, he claimed, an extraordinary number of ailments from pimples to cancer. So was created the myth of masturbatory insanity, a popular craze that enveloped Europe and the United States from the nineteenth century until recent years. Believing that children would scramble their brains through "self-abuse," an American physician, Graham, developed a type of wheat that, when eaten by children, would reduce their youthful experimentation. So was born the Graham cracker! Not to be outdone, Kellogg, famous for his sanitorium in Battle Creek, Michigan, invented another food, also designed to reduce the libidinous wandering of children's hands. And today, youngsters are still encouraged to eat breakfast cereals not unlike the corn flakes Dr. Kellogg served to the residents of his sanitorium (see Bullough, 1974 and Szasz, 1970, for reviews of this material). Even the profound Dr. Freud was taken in by the feared epidemic of masturbation and claimed, early in his career, that it caused neuresthenia. Modern psychoanalysis doesn't like to talk about that.[4]

How are we to view these ancestors, who not only invented a new disease, but also its cure, which included an extraordinary number of sadistic devices to be placed on children's genitals, clitoridectomies, incarceration, castration, and psychoanalysis? We can look at them as a momentary aberration, a glitch in the progress of science, or just as some cranky old men. But I think we are not so different from them. We can so easily see how misguided they were, so high in their motives, but so harmful to their patients. Perhaps the iatrogenic disorders caused by them in their time are not different from the iatrogenic disorders we cause today.

It is time, I think, to get morality out of psychological theory. Reviewing our reliance on DSM for diagnosis is one way to begin. Psychology should not condone or condemn behavior. That is a social function. I have not observed that psychologists have any greater wisdom about moral behavior than the population at large. Nor am I aware of any doctoral program with a course in morality and ethics, such topics having been purged years ago as vestiges of mentalism and the embarrassing philosophical roots of psychology. Our task is to understand the variables that contribute to making, in this case, one form of sexual activity more probable than another. It is my belief that both moral behavior and psychological knowledge will benefit from allowing each its due, and by getting psychoanalysts out of the business of being moral philosophers.

NOTES

1. It is extraordinary to note how long Rush's diagnoses have persisted in psychiatric circles. The first edition of DSM (1952) includes the following as mental illnesses: pathological mendacity, syphilophobia, vagabondage, untruthfulness, asocial trends, misanthropism, and cruelty (Silverstein, 1976/1977). By the time DSM II was published (1968), these afflictions, except for being "asocial," were downgraded from mental illnesses themselves to being symptoms of other mental disorders.

2. Abortion after quickening was already illegal. It was the belief at the time that a living soul entered the fetus only after quickening. For many people, including religious leaders, abortion before quickening was not a moral issue.

3. See McNeil (1976) for a good review of the historical Catholic teachings on homosexuality.

4. Marcus and Francis (1975) make every attempt to redeem Freud's anti-masturbation attitude and ignore the historical influences upon him, but their logic is tortuous because the position is absurd. Stekel (1950) was ahead of his time, maintaining a positive view of masturbation and all sexuality.

REFERENCE NOTES

1. American Psychiatric Association. (1973, December 15). Press release.

2. Wilson. B. (1972). *Memorandum to committee on nomenclature of the American Psychiatric Association: Should homosexuality be in the A. P. A. nomenclature.* New York, Gay Activist Alliance.

REFERENCES

American Psychiatric Association. (1952). *Diagnostic and statistical manual of mental disorders.* Washington, DC: APA.

American Psychiatric Association. (1968). *Diagnostic and statistical manual of mental disorders* (2nd ed.). Washington, DC: APA.

American Psychiatric Association. (1980). *Diagnostic and statistical manual of mental disorders* (3rd ed.). Washington, DC: APA.

Bancroft, J. (1974). *Deviant sexual behavior: Modifications and assessment.* London: Oxford University Press.

Barker-Benfield, B. (1975). Sexual surgery in late nineteenth century America. *International Journal of Health Services, 2,* 279–298.

Bayer, R. (1981). *Homosexuality and American psychiatry.* New York: Basic Books.

Begelman, D. A. (1977). Homosexuality: The ethical challenge: Paper 3. *Journal of Homosexuality, 2,* 213–219.

Bell, A. P., & Weinberg, M. S. (1978). *Homosexualities: A study of diversity among men and women.* New York: Simon and Schuster.

Bieber, I., Dain, H. J., Dince, P. R., Drellich, M. G., Grand, H. G. Gundlach, R. H., Kremer, M. W., Rifkin, A. H., Wilber, C. B., Bieber, T. B. (1962). *Homosexuality: A study of male homosexuals.* New York: Basic Books.

Bullough, V. (1974). Homosexuality and the medical model. *Journal of Homosexuality, 1,* 99–110.

Conrad, P., & Schneider, J. W. (1980). *Deviance and medicalization: From badness to sickness.* St. Louis: C. V. Mosby.

Davison, G. C. (1977). Homosexuality: The ethical challenge: Paper 1. *Journal of Homosexuality, 2,* 195–204.

Feldman, M. P., & MacCulloch, M. J. (1971). *Homosexual behavior: Therapy and assessment.* New York: Pergamon Press.

Feldman, P. (1977). Helping homosexuals with problems: A commentary and a personal view. *Journal of Homosexuality, 2,* 241–250.

Foucault, M. (1973). *Madness and civilization: A history of insanity in the age of reason.* (R. Howard, trans.) New York: Vintage/Random House.

Green, R. (1972). Homosexuality as a mental illness. *International Journal of Psychiatry, 10,* 77–98.

Halleck, S. L. (1971). *The politics of therapy.* New York: Science House Inc.

Hatterer, L. J. (1970). *Changing homosexuality in the male.* New York: McGraw Hill.

Holyroyd, J. C. & Brodsky, A. M. (1977). Psychologists' attitudes and practices regarding erotic and nonerotic physical contact with patients. *American Psychologist, 32,* 847–849.

Marcus, I. M. & Francis, J. J. (1975). *Masturbation from infancy to senescence.* New York: International University Press.

Marmor, J. (Ed.). (1965). *Sexual inversion: The multiple roots of homosexuality.* New York: Basic Books.

McNeil, J. (1976). *The church and the homosexual.* Kansas City: Sheed Andrews and McMeel.

Medical Aspects of Human Sexuality. (1977). Sexual survey #4: Current thinking on homosexuality, *11*(2), 110–111.

Mohr, J. C. (1978). *Abortion in America.* New York: Oxford University Press.

Money, (1977). J. Paraphilias. In J. Money & H. Musaph (Eds.), *Handbook of sexology.:* Elsevier/ North Holland Biomedical Press.

Money, J. (1981). Paraphilias: Phyletic origins of erotosexual dysfunction. *International Journal of Mental Health, 10*(2), 75–109.

Popper, K. P. (1959). *The logic of scientific discovery.* Toronto: University of Toronto Press.

Rosen, G. (1968). *Madness in society.* New York: Harper and Row.

Sedgwick, P. (1973). Illness—Mental and otherwise. *Hastings Center Studies,* V.1, No.3, p.27.

Silverstein, C. (1976/1977). Even psychiatry can profit from its past mistakes. *Journal of Homosexuality, 2,* 153–158.

Silverstein, C. (1977). Homosexuality: The ethical challenge: Paper 2. *Journal of Homosexuality, 2,* 205–212.

Socarides, C. W. (1975). *Beyond sexual freedom.* New York: Quadrangle (The New York Times Book Co.).

Stekel W. (1950). *Auto-eroticism: A psychiatric study in onanism and neurosis.* New York: Limelight.

Szasz, T. S. (1970). *The manufacture of madness.* New York: Delta Books.

Therapeutic Implications of Viewing Sexual Identity in Terms of Essentialist and Constructionist Theories

John Hart, MA

Sheffield City Polytechnic

ABSTRACT. One of the most challenging developments in recent historical studies and in empirical research in sociology has been constructionist
theories relating to "sexual personalities." The "constructionist" view is
that sexual identity is labile and can be therapeutically modified. In clinical
work, this has presented an alternative view of the development of social
sex-role and sexual orientation. Previously, views of sexual identity as a
fixed personal characteristic (the "essentialist" view) provided clinicians
with ways of treating psychologically distressed people either by transsexual conversion or aversion therapy. This article reviews some implications of "constructionist" and "essentialist" theory. It describes the
author's clinical attempts to present constructionist views to clients who
are in conflict about their sexual orientation and social sex-role. The article concludes that constructionist therapy has not taken into account clinical evidence that clients may adhere to "essentialist" beliefs.

This article is written from a particular clinical and therapeutic
perspective: that theory should inform practice and that practice should
critique, modify, correct, and create theory. In my own clinical research
and practice I have specialized in problems of social sex-role and sexual
orientation. As De Cecco (1981) pointed out, although these two aspects
of sexual identity are often, in clinical discussions, linked together, it is
important to consider social sex-role and sexual orientation as potentially
independent. Moreover, sexual orientation should be considered as three
dimensions: physical sexual activity, interpersonal affection, and erotic
fantasies.

John Hart is Principal Lecturer in Social Work at his institution in Sheffield, England, and a
therapist. He is co-author of *The Theory and Practice of Homosexuality* (London, 1981), and author
of a forthcoming (1984) book entitled *So You Think You Are Attracted to the Same Sex?* Requests for
reprints should be addressed to the author, Department of Applied Social Studies, Sheffield City
Polytechnic, Pond Street, Sheffield S11 NB, England.

This view of sexual identity inevitably leads us to a consideration of the current theoretical debate on "essentialist" versus "constructionist" views of an individual's sexual development (see Figure 1). I appreciate Plummer's (1981) statement that

> in the main, essentialists are clinicians who, whilst recognizing that homosexuality is an essence, would like to change the homosexual back into a heterosexual. Likewise, constructionists are sociologists who, whilst recognizing that homosexuality is a historical invention, agree that gay self-definitions have played a very positive role . . . whilst the label is needed now, it will ultimately be eliminated. (p. 108)

FIGURE 1.

THERAPEUTIC IMPLICATIONS OF ESSENTIALIST AND CONSTRUCTIONIST THEORIES

Theories	Therapeutic Implications
"ESSENTIALIST" THEORIES	
"Born that way"	Acceptance of "condition" Possibility of future biological manipulation
Psychoanalytic theory	Corrective Treatment to develop heterosexual personality
Sociobiological explanations of social sex-role or sexual orientation	Adjustment to sexual identity (surgical reassignment, social or psychological therapy)
"CONSTRUCTIONIST" THEORIES	
"Labeling" theory	Acceptance of deviant role as valid
Political theory/sexual choice	Political action/self help, identity support groups, consciousness - raising Reassignment to opposite biological sex Adjustment to a normative or deviant sex role
Historical invention of sexual categorization	Consciousness-raising Social therapy to accept notion of a 'labile' sexual identity

However, as both theoretician and clinician, I want to examine the possibilities of integrating constructionist theory with practice in dealing with problems of sexual identity.

The practical importance of the constructionist view of "sexual identities" is elucidated by considering the limitations of "essentialist" models alongside the evidence of 35 years of sexology. Researchers from Kinsey to Masters and Johnson have shown that people's sexual behavior reflects a diversity that cannot be explained by essentialist theories. Further, recent theoretical writings suggest that bisexuality encompasses an "invisible majority" of adults. MacDonald (1981), for example, has looked at the major studies of homosexuals and concluded that they have included many bisexuals, resulting in scientifically inaccurate reporting of individuals' erotic, affectional, and behavioral attractions.

In theory then, we are moving away from viewing people as having fixed sexual characters—heterosexual, bisexual, transvestite, transsexual, or homosexual. Such identities can instead be viewed as creations of the interaction between an individual and society at historically specific moments. We have elsewhere considered the development and maintenance of sexual orientation as a "choice" composed of many factors in an individual's life experience (Hart, 1981). However, we can also ask what the practical implications are of such theorizing about the potential lability of sexual identity.

To a large extent, people live in a world that is deterministically explained to and by them. The forces of culture and socialization are generally rendered invisible by the consensus ideology in both the United Kingdom and North America. These forces also affect "deviants" themselves who, despite the speculations of earlier theorists, are brought up in much the same way as those who are not so labeled. For example, Spada (1979, p. 274) reported this about gay men: "Most of the respondents stated either that there was 'no reason' that they were gay or that they were born that way." Similarly, sex-role behavior is seen as closely linked to aggressive "instincts" in men and mothering "instincts" in women.

In my clinical experience I have met 14-year-olds who assert that the reason for their homosexuality is "I just am," and older men who object to my using terms such as "coming out" because "it implies someone wasn't *that way* all along." Such individuals are describing much more than their sexual orientation; they are saying that they have come to know themselves as they "truly are." A man in his late 60s described his previous 40 years of heterosexual married life as "not really being myself." It had taken the death of his wife and tea-room sex to show him "who he was." A post-operative male-to-female transsexual, with whom I had been working in one-to-one therapy, had made many attempts at suicide, but later was surer that she wanted to live. On considering her future with some satisfaction, she stated: "In 30 or 40 years I'll die, but I'll die as I should have been born: a woman."

Despite these essentialist beliefs of patients, I believe that clinicians should take constructionist theories seriously. To do so provides people with a personal and political history of their lives that emphasizes the "choices" they have made—consciously or not. It also identifies the restrictions and stigmatizing events that they have experienced. It provides a model that is outward-looking rather than introspective and enables people to see their individual reactions as part of an experience they can share with others.

Let us look at the possible ways in which a clinician can respond to the "essentialist" beliefs of clients. First, the clinician may agree with such beliefs; many therapists see sexual identity as socially or psychically determined. They view individuals who are ill-at-ease with their sexual identity as being in conflict with their true selves and as needing a reduction in guilt or an increase in self-assertiveness. Other clinicians might see deviant sex-role behaviors, identities, or sexual orientations as part of an individual's psychological defense against the anxieties associated with attempting to conform to normative role behavior or the heterosexual orientation. Bieber (1965), for example, suggested that homosexuals choose to love a person of the same sex because of fear of the opposite sex. Such views merge into viewing the bisexual and homosexual orientations as involving pathological sex-role behavior. Socarides (1979), for example, writes of the adult male homosexual who "constantly yearns and searches for masculinity and, by engaging in homosexual acts, incorporates the male partner and his penis, thus 'strengthening' himself" (p. 258). Such clinical theorizing can form the basis for therapy that sees homosexual or atypical sex-role behavior as an acting out of early family conflicts and requires the patient to cease "acting out" and to develop insight into her or his "condition."

The essentialist beliefs can also be examined by the clinician from the point of view of role theory. We can, with the client, ask Plummer's (1975, p. 137) question: "Why, when so many people are potentially available for homosexual experiences and identification, do so few enter stable homosexual roles?" This may be extremely helpful for those who believe they are victims of some biological or psychological quirk and are thereby destined for a life of short-lived relationships and general unhappiness. Role theory can add a flexibility to people's view of themselves which, at best, may help them take responsibility for their lives.

Essentialist beliefs are also endorsed in the gay media, as illustrated by a letter I received after a gay newspaper reported on my theory of "choice" in sexual orientation. "Such a concept," the writer informed me, would "do great harm to the cause of sexual liberation and confuse young people who were already in conflict about their 'natural' homosexual drives." This opinion is explained by constructionist theory. A category can be seen as enabling: "At my first gay disco I breathed a big sigh and felt, 'I'm home; these are my people.' "

However, categorization also leads to stigma, discrimination and perhaps a narrowing of options for a future in which the sex-role sterotypes may change and relationships between men and women may not include their current inequalities. In such a future, sexual orientation could be relatively unimportant in defining individuals, enabling them to engage in relationships with both the opposite and the same sex. Indeed, those not doing so might be seen as having very specific phobias. Young teenagers now in counseling could grow into such a world; to limit them to interest in only one biological sex may not prepare them for future adult roles.

There is a fourth approach for the clinician to essentialist beliefs: using the concept of false consciousness. Nowhere is the belief in the essentiality of male and female sex-role behavior so firmly held as it is by people who believe they are "transsexuals." Let us consider a hypothetical situation in which someone decided after 40 years to change sexes, socially and surgically, in order to live as a person of the opposite biological sex. This change was desired not because of dissatisfaction with the present anatomy, but as a "political choice." It would be difficult to imagine any psychiatrist or medical specialist taking such a request seriously. The would-be transsexuals must themselves believe and convince professionals that they cannot be fulfilled as human beings without changing the body to fit the mind (or soul). One of the most direct challenges to a belief in a fixed sexual identity is found in Raymond's (1980) analysis of transsexualism, which uses the insights of radical feminism and the work of Thomas Szasz (e.g., 1970, 1974) to challenge the medical and moral view of male-to-female sex change. As an alternative to surgery and psychotherapy, Raymond offers a prescription—consciousness-raising groups for men who wish to be socially and surgically reassigned:

> Given peer encouragement to transcend cultural definitions of both masculinity and femininity, *without* changing one's body, persons considering transsexualism might not find it necessary to resort to sex-conversion surgery. (p. 183)

Raymond's position is that surgical reassignment involves a mutilation of "being." She believes consciousness-raising can provide a clinical alternative by challenging essentialist notions of sex-role behavior in the transsexual. Questions remain about its usefulness in problems of sexual orientation. The concept of the lability of sexual orientation is perhaps more familiar to those who work with people who have been married or otherwise partnered with the opposite sex and who, after a period of time, come to see their sexual orientation as other than heterosexual.

Greg, age 30, contacted me via a help line. He was a well-respected social worker with high professional standards. Ten years previously, while he had been in college he had married his childhood girlfriend. His marriage had been monogamous and his sexual relationship satisfactory. The couple had two boys, ages four and six. Greg remembered having erotic feelings toward men since he was 14, but said he was inhibited from acting them out. Shortly after the birth of his second son, he had begun driving up and down urban motorways, vaguely hoping to pick up a man. He saw himself as bisexual.

When I introduced him to a self-help group, he was initially disappointed, wanting to find a male sexual partner immediately. This is not uncommon for people who see themselves as having "dammed up" their homosexual erotic response, never translating these feelings into behavior and relationships. He then entered a period of intense homosexual activity, which caused him only minimum guilt and anxiety. This concentrated homosexual activity may occur at any age for homosexuals, whenever they first come out, although for heterosexuals it has traditionally been seen as a youthful phenomenon. Greg was sufficiently flexible in his view of sex-role behavior not to have to contend with fears about "taking the woman's role." This is by no means a universal freedom. One of my clients, who had previously been involved only in heterosexual relationships, when he discovered that he enjoyed taking the "passive" role in anal intercouse, told me that he worried he might develop as other of my clients, male-to-female transsexuals.

Frequently, however, people like Greg find that the problems of including homosexual behavior as part of their sexual identity are social rather than psychological. It is often easier for men than women to lead "double lives" because of economic resources. For both sexes, however, the problems of monogamy, trust and stigma, and emotional and physical energy, interact to insure that they usually alternatively enter "gay" and "straight" relationships. If they are married, either the heterosexual relationship is abandoned or homosexual relationships are severely restricted.

For Greg, the therapeutic task was not to provide a view of sexuality as labile, but to help him create space in his marriage for both his wife and himself to have sexual relationships outside of the home while still shouldering the responsibilities of raising young children. However, Greg's view of sex-roles was vital if the marriage was to go on being fulfilling for *both* partners. Over time, other relationships may become more demanding. The consequences are no different from those experienced by people who seek heterosexual relationships outside of their primary one. If dependent children are involved, however, the law may well discriminate in custody cases against someone involved in a homosexual relationship.

I am suggesting that certain individuals are able to have both homosexual and heterosexual relationships without the conflicts that may be associated with an "essentialist" view of sex-roles and sexual orientation. I have indicated that the clinician's job is to provide social acceptance. However, the psychological variable is how flexible the person's view of social sex-role can be.

The attitude of the patient's partner is also important. Greg and his wife intended to share child care. This was partly accomplished by sharing a new home with another heterosexual couple, who were also social workers, and their children. The new living situation provided Greg's wife with more time alone and she began demanding Greg's presence in the home. The "weight" of heterosexual family life compelled Greg to decide that he would not be able to go out to gay meeting places and have sexual relations with men. Thus he soon after decided, "I will have to repress this side of myself." Greg therefore returned to a slightly altered form of exclusively heterosexual family life, at least temporarily.

Perhaps the test of the constructionist theory of a labile sexual orientation is in moving from homosexual to heterosexual encounters. One of my patients, Henry, was 30 before he had a sexual relationship with anyone. His first heterosexual experience occurred in his late 30s, after he had experienced a number of relationships with men. He decided to experiment with women, since he found both sexes attractive. He felt, although he was slightly more erotically attracted to men, that heterosexual relationships were more socially rewarding. Henry was fortunate in having a close female friend who encouraged him to have sex with her on what was virtually a systematic desensitization basis. He continued to enjoy relationships with men, and this dual pattern suited his needs.

Henry saw himself as bisexual. Unlike Greg, he did not have to manage his homosexual relationships carefully to insure that his primary relationship was not threatened. It is the social considerations, rather than the psychological ones, that enable people to move in and out of both heterosexual and homosexual relationships without a major threat to their sexual identity. This is not possible for larger numbers of people because of the stigma that is attached to homosexual relationships.

Simon's case shows the way in which constructionist views can help people deal with social stigma. He was brought up in a liberal, educated, and reasonably affluent middle class family. At school he was a loner, unable or unwilling to take on what was seen as the appropriate sex-role behavior. "I just felt different at school, liking things the girls used to like, hating football. Terribly stereotypical differences, I'm afraid to say." He saw his home as a safe place where he could create his own fantasy world, giving his large extended family imperial titles and populating a flower garden with snapdragons which were given royal names. From his early teens he was called "queer," "poof," "woman," and he began to associate these names with "being a homosexual." He added his early fears of being unacceptable on to the fear of being homosexual, which he saw as "a horrendous deviance." Simon felt he could be heterosexual: "If I tried hard enough. Every few months I would have purges. I would decide not to look at men or think about them as I had been doing since I was sixteen." He was so unhappy that he "identified with the aggressor" by becoming outrageously camp, while also joining the Army Officer Training Corps. He sometimes discussed homosexuality negatively so that others would not really believe he was homosexual.

Simon came into therapy wanting to be rid of his homosexuality, which he saw as overwhelming. I helped him to see that his self-perceived differences were part of his personality and that, rather than being predestined to be a homosexual, he could choose his sexual orientation. The important thing was his self-acceptance. As his understanding increased, so did his conflicts. Because he was obsessed with outward appearances, he decided that if being a homosexual was itself not the problem, then he could never be acceptable as a homosexual because he could not attain the macho look currently fashionable for male homosexuals. He was then obsessed about developing muscles, attempting to improve his physique. I tried to convince him that his obsession with becoming a popular gay male sex object was confusing sex-role behavior with sexual orientation, and that all this was overlaid by a basic nonacceptance of himself.

I want to emphasize how this "therapeutic pushing outwards" was for Simon a treatment strategy preferable to delving into his early family conflicts. I also encouraged him to talk about his heterosexual orientation, in terms of his interpersonal relationships with women, his erotic fantasies, and his fears that he would not be successful in heterosexual acts. He began to see that the forbidden, different, and apparently overwhelming aspects of homosexual relationships were what made it for him the "right choice" at that moment in his life. He stated: "Despite the tremendous disadvantages, it became almost a delight to be what society saw as sexually deviant. It made it all the more appealing."

Although he had been staunchly conservative in politics, Simon developed a different political view of sexual choice. In a self-help group, I was surprised to hear him inform a young gay Christian that being gay meant challenging Christian ideology. Simon believed Christianity endorsed certain family and authority forms, while homosexual relationships provided an alternative egalitarian society that enabled people to overcome barriers of class, sex, and age. Although he still had some fantasy about the gay world's contribution to human progress, Simon had managed to move from the belief that he was a "victim of nature" to a positive assertion of his homosexual identity. I believe that consciousness raising was enormously helpful in his personal therapy. The alternative psychodynamic approach might have made him less able to value himself, although theoretically it could have lead to the achievement of a heterosexual orientation.

Simon's case points to the importance of the political stance of the therapist who adopts a constructionist approach. If he or she believes that individuals are not biologically or psychically destined to be heterosexual or homosexual, the therapist is clearly placed in the role of a moral agent. Do we encourage human diversity or conformity? Traditionally, a "client-centered" approach has been the answer. But what about those situations in which the therapist believes that false consciousness is the client's central presenting problem? Can people who are exhibiting, and in some ways glorifying, sex-role rigidity, such as transvestites or transsexuals, really be encouraged to find what they see as their "true selves" if this means radical surgical and psychological readjustment? If not, can they be helped to understand and correct their false consciousness?

I will describe my work with a post-operative, transsexual as an illustration of the power of sex role rigidities in our culture, as well as the limitations of consciousness-raising therapy. Michael was born in 1945 in Scotland. In 1979 he had two operations in order to become "Wendy," having dressed and behaved as a women for just 14 months before "the operations." Previously, Michael had a long history of medical treatment; from his childhood he had mastoids, perforations of the ear, and breathing problems, which meant that he was hospitalized much of the time during the first ten years of his life. He felt different, an outsider from his family, who lived in a rough, working-class city.

He had begun to cross-dress at the age of nine, and by the time he was ten he was called "poof" and "queer" at school. At 11, he was "raped by a Scout Troop leader," and "Wendy," as a small baby, was born inside his head. Two years later his stepfather began to frequently sexually abuse him. During adolescence, "Wendy' "grew into a young girl" and Michael withdrew into a "world of books," encouraged by a friendship with a female school librarian. "Wendy" reported that he enjoyed then a "vast educational improvement," except in male-dominated activities (e.g., woodwork, metalwork):

> I did not participate in physical exercises. I had few friends of my own age. I hero-worshipped an older boy but was confused by the feelings and the name-calling. I began to think of myself as a woman but, because of religious and educational teaching [she is a Roman Catholic], I thought this meant homosexuality. I gradually became completely withdrawn.

When Michael was 16 his mother died, after having a stormy second marriage. By the time he was 18, Michael had experienced his first heterosexual intercourse. He also sought psychiatric help for "problems in relating to people." By the age of 21, Michael was diagnosed as an alcoholic and received inpatient psychiatric treatment. A year later, he began a long relationship with a woman who was to have two children by him and, later, to marry him, accept his cross-dressing, and finally divorce him after supporting his surgical change over to "Wendy." Michael had this to say about his former wife: "She was very supportive. She was with me when they came with the trolley to take me to the theatre for the surgical reassignment. Michael, her husband, went off and Wendy came back."

Michael/Wendy was unable to keep a job and continued to receive psychiatric help. Between the ages of 25 and 30, Michael met transvestites and transsexuals and it was then he decided that a sex change was necessary to "kill off Michael." He was a heterosexual male with conservative sexual and social mores who, given his conventional appearance, could never understand why he was called names or why men made sexual advances to him. He remained very fearful. He became a day-patient at a psychiatric hospital. "Drugs became part of my life. I overdosed once in a while."

Although Michael saw his wife's pregnancies as "proof of my manhood, it was no good—the image of 'Wendy' grew stronger." In 1977 he met a psychotherapist who tried to reconstruct his identity as a male; the therapist accepted Michael's sex-role behavior differences and encouraged him to tell his wife. This therapeutic initiative resulted in more acting out by Michael and increased his desire to change sexes.

After his second reassignment operation he

> decided to die as a woman. Life became confused. [I] tried to hold on but couldn't. Michael returned and I went completely berserk . . . more and more drugs . . . at one time I thought I was four people . . . I was frequently hospitalized. My friends agreed to kill me but this failed, and I ended up in intensive care. Finally I met a sympathetic psychiatrist who referred me to a therapeutic community.

When I met Wendy and offered to work with her to help her understand her struggles for a sexual identity, she replied, "I'd rather die." But later she asked to begin working on her identity problems. (I prefer to describe the situation at this time as an "identity vacuum.") Having failed to come to terms with problems of sex-role and sexual orientation, despite every kind of psychiatric assistance, she was allowed to "become a woman" without the usual role transition period. The fact that "Michael," whom

Wendy saw as "bad," did not disappear under the surgeon's knife confronted her with the prospect of personal annihiliation.

Wendy and I began, with many setbacks ("Michael's" deep, working-class voice would take over when Wendy was under stress) to build up her sexual identity. This meant facing the implications of her earlier sexual experiences as a man. Wendy made some progress in accepting that (s)he had been in conflict with a homosexual identity, and this led to my trying to link sexual orientation with a general and critical view of traditional masculine sex-role behavior. I suggested that she could identify with gay persons, not because she essentially was one, but because of their criticism of traditional sex-roles. I suggested that her past experience had been with men who took on violent and oppressive sex-role stereotypes. This interpretation was difficult for her to accept. Anything that smacked of feminist criticism was written off by Wendy (I'm not a women's libber myself") as "communist propaganda." She read, or rather looked at, Raymond's (1980) book, which she picked up from my bookshelf, in the same spirit.

There was a thin line between challenging her beliefs and respecting her "defenses." For example, her view was the traditional one that sex was only for procreation. Although I sometimes had to refer her to her spiritual advisor, I did offer alternative views of Christian teaching on sexual mores. This did seem to free her to engage in sexual relationships. I would also give advice: After she brought a new boyfriend to see me, one who "had in the past been gay," she confided that intercourse with him was very painful and she had been bleeding. I suggested that she use a lubricant. When she said that was only for homosexual men, I was able to inform her of its proper use in heterosexual as well as homosexual intercourse. I also encouraged her to see her surgeon, who provided her with a dilator for her surgically constructed vagina.

Wendy is currently enjoying the longest period of time in her life free from regular psychiatric treatment. She has begun to enjoy her sexuality, although in much the same way as drag queens I have known. She is adopting a reflexive approach to her situation, realizing that Wendy is a social rather than a surgical construction, and that aspects of the male role are still going to be with her. Perhaps that is the most difficult task for Wendy—to realize that "Michael" is part of her and, indeed, that the woman she wishes to become is based on the man she never allowed herself to be.

This case history may show both the opportunities and the limitations of consciousness-raising for people who are literally "wounded refugees" of a sexist society. It is a society that is "transsexualgenic." My view is that it is not the task of clinicians to attempt to change that society by using people who are already overwhelmed by its contradictions. I am aware that Raymond (1980) and others are also criticizing the medical and psychiatric establishment, but such professionals are frequently subjected to much pressure from people like Wendy who demand that transsexual surgery be provided, literally as a life-saving measure.

CONCLUSION

This article has been about the possibilities of moving from an "essentialist" to an "constructionist" base in clinical practice. I have described my own attempts to test the theory in practice by using role theory and consciousness-raising. For some people, their experience of social sex-roles enables them to see sexual orientation as labile. For others, it is possible to introduce constructionist dialogues into individual or group therapy and, by doing so, to give them an analysis of their situation that can free them from tortured introspection. I conclude, however, that the critics who dismiss the belief in a fixed sexual identity have failed to see that it is held by many people who come for therapy. The concept of false consciousness cannot be applied to someone who has undergone such a radical life event as surgical sex reassignment. It is possible for some people to choose to take on transvestite, heterosexual, homosexual, or transsexual roles, but for others, no such choice exists at a particular point in their lives. Wendy, for example, may see that she has been socially as well as surgically reassigned; indeed, it is important to her future for her to see herself as being in control of her own life. We cannot, however, move from this point back into her life history and *reconstruct* her identity in retrospect. Perhaps the professionals could have withheld surgery. But what had to be recognized was that "Michael" saw himself essentially as a woman.

This brings us to a position represented by Raymond—the ontological wholeness of chromosomal sex. Indeed, this could be seen as "the new essentialism," but it does point us away from the victims and back to what we may learn from the phenomenon of transsexualism and about the real sex differences between women and men. As clinicians, we should conclude that neither the belief in a fixed nor in a labile sexual identity does justice to people's experience of their sexual identities. To argue that either of these positions is "true" may be good politics, but it is bad therapy, and inadequate sexology.

REFERENCES

Bieber, I. (1965). Clinical aspects of male homosexuality. In J. Marmor (Ed.), *Sexual inversion: The multiple roots of homosexuality.* New York: Basic Books.
De Cecco, J. P. (1981). Definition and meaning of sexual orientation. *Journal of Homosexuality, 6,* 51-67.

Hart, J., & Richardson, D. (1981). *The theory and practice of homosexuality.* London & Boston: Routledge & Kegan Paul.

MacDonald, A. P. (1981). Bisexuality: Some comments on research and theory. *Journal of Homosexuality, 6.*

Plummer, K. (1975). *Sexual stigma: An interactionist account.* London & Boston: Routledge & Kegan Paul.

Plummer, K. (1981). Going gay: Identities, life cycles and lifestyles in the male gay world. In Hart, J. & Richardson, D. (Eds.), *The theory and practice of homosexuality.* London & Boston: Routledge & Kegan Paul.

Raymond, J. G. (1980). *The transsexual empire.* London: The Women's Press.

Socarides, C. (1979). The psychoanalytic theory of homosexuality with special reference to therapy. In I. Rosen (Ed.), *Sexual Deviation* (2/e). Oxford: Oxford University Press.

Spada, J. (1979). *The Spada report.* New York: Signet Books.

Szasz, T. S. (1970). *The manufacture of madness: A comparative study of the inquisition and the mental health movement.* New York: Harper & Row.

Szasz, T. S. (1974). *The myth of mental illness.* New York: Harper & Row.

Conceptualizations of Homosexual Behavior Which Preclude Homosexual Self-Labeling

Joel D. Hencken, PhD (cand.)

University of Michigan

ABSTRACT. Our culture presents people with a problematic pair of messages: (1) engaging in homosexual behavior makes a person a homosexual, and (2) homosexuality is bad. In this context, maintenance of self-esteem, sexual/affectional satisfaction, and coherent identity requires some intricate psychological footwork. This article describes a variety of common conceptualizations of "homosexual behavior" which permit the individual to avoid the stigma of homosexual self-labeling. It is suggested that the "accuracy" of these constructions is less important than the appropriate doubt they cast on our widely held, but psychologically inadequate, concepts of sexual orientation.

Homosexual self-labeling in our culture involves ascribing to oneself a trait which is culturally devalued, i.e., stigmatized (Goffman, 1974/1963). As a result, people usually attempt alternative constructions of their feelings, fantasies, and behavior, and only self-label as homosexual if and when such alternatives cannot be made to "stick." It is tempting—and, indeed, it is common among therapists and many gay activists—to describe such alternative constructions as necessarily defensive in nature, based on some objectified definition of what is homosexual. I will refrain from such a global designation here for two reasons.

First, the symbolic interactionists (Hart & Richardson, 1981; Plummer, 1975) have argued rather persuasively that something is sexual only

Joel Hencken is a psychotherapist in Boston, MA, and a doctoral candidate in clinical psychology at the University of Michigan. He was Clinical Director of the Homophile Community Health Service (Boston) from 1979-1981. Currently, he serves as editor of the *Association of Lesbian and Gay Psychologists Newsletter*, and as a member of the editorial board of the *Journal of Homosexuality*. He is co-author of "Coming Out as an Aspect of Identity Formation" (*Gay Academic Union Journal: Gai Saber*, 1977) and author of "Homosexuality and Psychoanalysis: Toward a Mutual Understanding" (*American Behavioral Scientist*, 1982). Requests for reprints should be addressed to the author, 14 Myrtle Street, Jamaica Plain, MA 02130.

Presented at the Sixth World Congress of Sexology, May 1983, Washington, D.C. This article is based on a section of "Homosexual Identities: An Exploration of Issues," Prelim paper in clinical psychology, The University of Michigan, 1982.

53

insofar as it is personally and socially defined as such. Second, I take seriously the particularities of our historical period, especially its reification of sexual *behavior* into sexual *orientation* and its limitation of sexual orientation to two, or at most three, categories (heterosexual, homosexual, bisexual). If, in other words, it could confidently be claimed that every person is or is not a homosexual but may or may not, for a variety of reasons, be aware of it at any given point in his or her life, then we could for each person posit a "real" sexual orientation and call nonrecognition of it a defense, mediated in most cases by a combination of motivated and simple ignorance. But this claim is itself quite dubitable. Indeed, it is one of our purposes to keep it an open question; for while it is clearly part of our cultural belief-system, it is hardly susceptible of empirical proof at present and, as the interactionists argue, it is also theoretically suspect. As a result, we will simply describe some of the psychological constructions some people make of experiences which lead other people to self-label as homosexual (see Cass, 1979).

(a) *I was drunk.* The attribution of socially proscribed behavior to drug-altered states is so widespread as to require little elaboration. In his play *The Boys in the Band,* Crowley (1968) calls the phenomenon the "Christ-was-I-drunk-last-night syndrome." Note that he also captures the attitude toward it of people who subsequently self-label as homosexual:

> The Christ-was-I-drunk-last-night syndrome. You know, when you made it with some guy in school and the next day when you had to face each other there was always a lot of shit-kicking crap about, "Man was I drunk last night! Christ, I don't remember a thing!" . . . . It has to do with immaturity. (p. 29) . . . . Yes, long before Justin or I or God only knows how many others *came out,* we used to get drunk and "horse around" a bit. You see, in the Christ-was-I-drunk-last-night syndrome, you really *are* drunk. That part of it is true. It's just that you also *do remember everything. /General laughter/* Oh God, I used to have to get loaded to go in a gay bar! (p. 30; italics his)

Cultural psychopharmacology has changed significantly in recent years, however, and today the description would have to be extended to include being "stoned" on marijuana, or "on" a variety of other common drugs—uppers, downers, hallucinogens, and sundry other psychotropics.

(b) *Just trade.* The "just trade" concept is common coin among hustlers and men who are "kept" by other, more affluent, men. It emphasizes that sex is being performed for money rather than for pleasure, although many people who employ this construction will reckon that the sexual release is a (perhaps minor) fringe benefit of this line of work. The hustlers very frequently do not regard themselves as homosexual, although they invariably regard their clients—even the heterosexually married ones—as such. In many cases, these men later self-label as homosexual. When they do, they regard the just-trade notion as a form of denial of their homosexuality, which they, subsequently, typically speak of as having been there all along, unacknowledged.

A significant number, however, stop hustling after a time and go on to more-or-less exclusively heterosexual lives. These men are likely to tacitly continue the just-trade construction of their past lives, particularly since there is rarely any external pressure to think further about it, and there is usually internal pressure *not* to. It may be noted that this population includes men who solicit both male and female customers during all or part of their hustling "careers" (see Plummer, 1975), and may or may not have boy- and/or girlfriends while hustling. Research at present is too preliminary to ascertain any reliable patterns as to who in this varied group will later self-label as homosexual. (See Hoffman, 1972.) Sometimes the just-trade construction is combined with:

(c) *I just "get done."* This phrase refers to a man who allows another man—frequently but not necessarily a paying customer—to touch, kiss, fellate, or masturbate him; or with whom he is the insertor in anal intercourse; or in front of whom he masturbates or performs other sexually provocative behaviors while the other man masturbates. The psychological emphasis is on the fact that he does not "reciprocate" the homosexual feelings of the other. This concept, illustrated in John Rechy's (1967) novel, *Numbers,* is central to the conscious regulation of self-esteem. A variant occurs among gay men as well: Rechy describes men who, while they see themselves as homosexual, achieve a sense of higher status by being the one who "gets done" rather than the one who "does" the other.

In this construction, then, homosexuality is defined by the particular role played in the sexual behavior. The definition typically conforms to the notion that only the receiver of the penis is a homosexual (this is also common in Latin subcultures and some cultures of antiquity: Boswell, 1980), although it may be more idiosyncratically defined, e.g., "I didn't come," or "I didn't feel anything." These constructions are frequently viewed by others with suspicion because it appears that homosexuality is deliberately defined in any way which will get the individual "off the hook." Most clinicians would doubtless opine that all such cases illustrate defensive distortion, but it is likely that people who employ this kind of construction are not all defending against quite the same thing. What seems most prominent for men who use this construction is the need to guard their sense of masculinity, since it is sometimes used by men who have already self-labeled as homosexual.

(d) *It's just physical.* This construction, as far as I know also a uniquely male one, explains, for example, the appearance of an erection in a same-sex context as due to physical stimulation but without sexual meaning. It is often stated aloud, with some embarrassment, and with considerable forced humor. For example, if a man is getting a professional massage at a gym, or two athletes are exchanging massages, the recipient may develop an erection which he explains in this fashion. It is interesting that this may be followed by the full range of explicitly sexual behaviors without major change in the psychological construction. However, when elaborate sex follows, the strategy is usually supplemented by others, e.g., "I just 'get done,'" or:

(e) *I was just horny.* Here the physical arousal is acknowledged at some point as having a sexual meaning, but it is attributed to a general condition of sexual deprivation and the homosexual context is dismissed as irrelevant. It may serve as an explanation for an erection and not lead to sexual activity, or only, say, to masturbation in private; or sex may ensue, but be regulated by a variety of "I just 'get done'"; or the man may engage in any kind of sexual behavior with the partner(s), but explain it by saying, "As long as I was horny and the other guy was there—why not?"

The actual sexual behaviors that accompany psychological constructions (d) and (e) depend in considerable measure, of course, on the other person as well. If he uses a complementary construction, is self-identified as homosexual or bisexual, is attractive, or is good at sexual persuasion, more is likely to happen. When it does, the next quartet of strategies may be employed:

(f) *I was just experimenting.* This construction is common in, but hardly limited to, undergraduate circles under the rubric of what is sometimes called "bisexual chic," where peer pressure for sexual experimentation may be considerable. The extent to which a person can engage in homosexual behavior and still call it "experimenting" varies across individuals and social circles. For one-time experiences, the construction is perhaps better called *I was just curious.*

It is interesting, however, that for some people the "experiment" may include many partners or occasions, or even a relationship of months or years. An illustration is in some of the discussions of Evelyn Waugh's (1945) *Brideshead Revisited,* where it is claimed that the characters were in love but not homosexual, and the relationship is construed as "just" part of the English process of growing up (D.E., 1982). Whether the construction is "legitimate" is usually determined by the individual only retrospectively, after a heterosexual or homosexual label is firmly adopted; observers tend, without benefit of any clearly articulated set of criteria, to make their judgments *en bloc.* While the sexual novice is probably more inclined to use the "experimenting" construction, those with more extensive sexual experience are more likely to say:

(g) *It's just for variety.* This construction is most familiar to the popular imagination in connection with wealthy, famous, powerful, or aristocratic people who have become jaded about nearly everything, including sex. It is, however, also used by more ordinary folk, who regard whatever homosexual behavior they engage in as the "spice of variety," and may or may not consider themselves bisexual. It may be supplemented by "I just 'get done,'" especially when it is psychologically necessary to control the role played in sex. It also may serve as a construction secondary to "It's just physical," to explain the move from sexual arousal to sexual activity. For men, when homosexual behavior is frequent, the person may also employ the following pair of constructions:

(h) *It's more available with guys.* This refers to the part of the gay male population for whom casual sexual encounters are frequent. Men—frequently heterosexually married—who do not self-label as homosexual, sometimes say that they would just as soon, or even prefer, to have casual sexual encounters with women, but find them less available—"Women always want a *relationship!*" or "Why bother keeping a mistress?" These men usually emphasize the lack of relationship in such sexual encounters as evidence that they are not homosexual. Some also seek other men who regard themselves as heterosexual or bisexual, calling self-labeled homosexuals "professional gays," whom they may regard with considerable contempt. "Personal" classified ads often specify, e.g., "MWM BB sks sim for ————," i.e., "married white male body-builder seeks similar for (specify sexual activity or euphemism such as 'mutual admiration' or 'physical sharing')."

(i) *Only another man/woman really knows how to please.* While this statement is made by people of both sexes, it appears more common for men when used in the process of *rejecting* a homosexual label. (It probably functions with equal frequency for men and women as a justification for homosexual self-labeling.) The common form of this construction is illustrated by a married man whose wife is either opposed to or, in his view, inadequate in performing fellatio; he may seek homosexual partners periodically when he wants this form of sexual satisfaction. Since it is obvious that there are women who are perfectly adept in this area, further explanation for seeking men is generally indicated. This construction seems to be based on the line of reasoning that other men will understand fellatio simply because they also have penises. While Masters and Johnson (1979) did indeed state that in their sample the gay partners were more sexually compatible than the heterosexuals, apparently providing some evidence for construction (i), the line of reasoning from physical similarity to better sexual technique is dubious. It seems equally plausible that practice and freedom from inhibition are the more relevant variables.

In any case, construction (i) may be invoked in such a way that the person might be talking about which auto mechanic gives the superior tune-up. The sexual activity may be very frequent, and guilt may or may not accompany it, but there are no avowed implications for sexual orientation.

(j) *It was just a phase/I was just a kid.* This construction is used retrospectively, often in conjunction with (d), (e), (f), and (h). It ascribes the homosexuality to a period in life which is either viewed as a special developmental stage (which, e.g., Sullivan, 1947, argues should *not* be called a normal "homosexual stage") or experienced as discontinuous with the present, and for which responsibility is either not felt or actively (i.e., defensively) denied. When elaborated, the discussion of this construction usually involves describing that period in the life cycle as light-years away and invoking generalizations like "You know how kids are," or "We didn't know what we were doing" (not in the sense of "I was drunk," but rather meaning "We didn't know it was *sex*"). "It was just a phase" is often associated with:

(k) *It was the only game in town.* This refers to what is generally called situational, as to be distinguished from preferential, homosexuality (see Marmor, 1980). It usually involves living in same-sex environments, e.g., boarding schools, the military, prison, or seminary. However, it is also used in reference to same-sex day schools and college fraternities or sororities, so the extent to which the opposite sex was objectively rather than psychologically unavailable varies from case to case.

Another important feature which subdivides the population using this construction is whether the person was fantasizing about the opposite sex during the homosexual activity. For persons vigorously rejecting homosexual self-labeling, information about heterosexual fantasies, if they were present, is usually volunteered as part of construction (k). If heterosexual fantasies were not present, the person either does not think of their relevance or else admits their absence only with reluctance when questioned specifically—often with the production of supplementary rationales, e.g., "I was drunk." In some cases, of course, a person who believes that lack of heterosexual fantasies is incriminating will simply lie and say that they were present.

(l) *I was seduced.* This construction attributes the occurrence of any homosexual episodes to the persuasive influence of the other person(s) involved. This is most commonly assumed to happen when the partner is older, sexually more experienced, or clearly homosexual, but this construction is also frequently used when the partner is an age-mate. It is often associated with constructions (a), (e), (h), and (j). Examples: "He got me drunk and put the make on me"; "He convinced me by saying 'Don't knock it if you haven't tried it' "; "He told me I was just being uptight and old-fashioned about sex"; etc. Sometimes the partner was just very persistent. And sometimes people aver, "I just couldn't say no," often referring to their affection or esteem for the partner, as well as their own perceived inability to be assertive.

It may be noted that "I was seduced" is frequently *not* issued as a *complaint*. The individual may recount the incident(s) with apparent or even avowed pleasure, yet attribute responsibility to the partner(s), e.g., "I'd never have had the guts to make the first move myself." Given the dearth of research, whether or not the individual subsequently self-labels as homosexual is not predictable from how the person consciously describes the incident(s) at the time. "I was seduced" is often associated with:

(m) *I didn't really like it.* Here the person may conceptualize the reasons for engaging in homosexual activities in a variety of ways, but avers that he or she is not homosexual because they were not particularly pleasurable. For one-time experiences this may be relatively unproblematic. The more interesting use of this construction is for repeated homosexual experiences, with one or more partners. Crowley (1968) has one of his characters rather caustically operationalize the validity criteria of this kind of construction as follows:

> One time, it's youth. Twice, a phase maybe. Several times, *you like it!* (p. 121; italics his)

This operationalization is probably not very different from the popular view of both gays and nongays, except when it refers either to oneself when one is rejecting a homosexual label, or to someone in whose heterosexuality one is emotionally invested, e.g., one's child or a famous person (see construction (f); Crew & Norton, 1974; D.E., 1982). Here is an excellent example of the social character of distinctions which are often alleged to be exclusively scientific in nature.

A final note on the "I didn't really like it" construction: Its employment—with respect to the very same events—varies over time, largely as a function of the individual's current sexual-orientation self-labeling and attitudes toward homosexuality. Both of these, in turn, are undoubtedly part-functions of the current attitudes in both the overall culture and the person's particular milieu. When it is psychologically and socially acceptable to have liked the homosexual experiences, at least some of them are more likely to be reported as having been enjoyable. Whether this is the unconscious becoming conscious or a retrospective falsification may be terribly difficult to ascertain.

The next two constructions form a pair insofar as they both refer to a specific relationship context. The first emphasizes the nature of the relationship, and the second the self-labeling implications of an avowed homosexual relationship:

(n) *Just fond friends.* This construction is used in two related ways: by participants in the relationship, and by observers of it.

For participants, it can be used under two sets of conditions: when there is explicitly sexual activity, and when there is not. The gist of this construction is that whatever happens in the relationship is solely a natural expression of the feelings of the participants for one another, and is without implications for either their sexual orientations or their feelings or behavior in other relationships.

If the construction is challenged, either by others or in the participants' own thinking, the presence or absence of explicit sexual behavior lends specific shape to the construction. For example, when present, explicit sex may be admitted but viewed as simply an expression of caring or closeness that was natural and unpremeditated at each occurrence; the person may consider it as in the same category as putting one's arm around a friend's shoulder when he or she is emotionally upset. The construction may also, of course, be supplemented by others, e.g., (a), (d), (e), (f), (g), (j), and (m).

If explicit sex is absent, but a generalized sensual aura surrounds the relationship, it is emotionally intense, and the participants spend an unusual amount of time together, or otherwise have lives that are clearly more intertwined than is the case in ordinary friendships, then the question turns on the issue of implicit or latent homosexuality. In this construction, the person avers that there is, so to say, no homosexual subtext. Indeed, people who employ "just fond friends" are likely to reject the existence of subtexts generally: Things simply are what they are, rather than what they "mean" (see Shapiro, 1965).

For observers, construction (n) stipulates where the burden of proof is to be placed when deciding whether either explicit or implicit homosexuality is present. That is, observers using "just fond friends" require explicit proof that the participants engage in overtly sexual relations or that unconscious homosexuality is present. This may take the form of rejecting altogether the notion of unconscious homosexuality as a psychodynamic foundation for friendship (see Fenichel, 1945; Hocquenghem, 1978/1972); or, somewhat paradoxically, it may involve acceptance of that notion as so universal that the existence of homosexuality in this particular relationship is made to seem unimportant because, after all, *all* same-sex relationships are in *some* sense homosexual.

(o) *I just love X.* This construction may involve an amplification of "just fond friends," where love, but not homosexuality, is avowed. It appears to be much more common for woman than men. For example, in the controversy about the posthumously published letters between Eleanor Roosevelt and Lorena Hickok (see Faber, 1980), many commentators took this view of the relationship, attributing even the references to physical touching as merely reflective of early-twentieth-century literary extravagance (see Crew & Norton, 1974). Many others preferred the "just fond friends" construction.

However, another form of this construction is where the relationship, but not the participants, is considered homosexual. A popular example is tennis champion Billie Jean King's affair with another woman, which made national news and about which King, who is heterosexually married, spoke in terms of having had a genuine lesbian affair, but not being a lesbian.

"I just love X" is actually more complicated than has been presented, for a person may say he or she was not homosexual even at the time, or is *no longer* homosexual. Here it need only be said that whether or not the person *says* they *changed* sexual orientation, or that they had a homosexual relationship despite being heterosexual, probably depends more on the politics of disclosure than on having an articulated, conscious theory of sexual orientation. Under present social conditions, it is very difficult to collect data which would speak to the historical accuracy of self-labeling at the time of the relationship. The important thing about construction (o) is that it is a way of circumventing, at least partially or temporarily, the culturally given conviction that two or three categories will cover the entire range of human sexual orientations.

(p) *I made a political decision to have a homosexual relationship.* This construction is virtually unique to women, and goes by the official title of "political lesbianism." It may be described briefly as a sexual relationship being attributed primarily to ideological convictions. While it may be supplemented by constructions (f), (g), (i), (m), (n), and (o), it tends at this historical moment to be given primary status when it is used at all. This construction is particularly interesting theoretically, for it is conspicuously based on the notion that sexual orientation is *chosen* rather than *discovered*—a distinction which appears to be sex-linked: Men tend to use the language of discovery, women the language of choice. Whether these are two ways of talking about the same process, or differences in language which reflect differences in process, is at present unknown. Indeed, it has received only scant research attention.

CONCLUSION

In our culture, everyone seems to have an ox in danger of being gored when it comes to sexual orientation. If a person is in some way admirable, gay people—like nations and other minorities (see Gay, 1978; Grunfeld, 1979)—often point to the person's homosexual experience by way of, as it were, laying claim to him or her. If the person is repellant, the discussion is likely to involve more stringent critera for their being "really gay." Many heterosexuals tend to reject as homosexual an undesirable person who has had any homosexual history, but will deny the significance, or even the existence, of the person's homosexuality if he or she is highly admired (see Crew & Norton, 1974, for examples in the literary world; and Tripp, 1975, more generally).

Scholarly discussion, of course, is by no means immune to such politics, although the arguments tend to be less raucous. Scientists, moreover, have the opportunity to use "objective" operational definitions, which cannot in principle be faulted, but which may produce troubling effects (see Davison, 1976, 1982; Hencken, 1982; Paul, Weinrich, Gonsiorek, & Hotvedt, 1982; Szasz, 1961). For example, Socarides (1978) has articulated a diagnostic category of "schizo-homosexuality" to describe people who are both homosexual and schizophrenic, and the American Psychiatric Association's new *DSM-III* lists "ego-dystonic homosexuality" as a disorder. Neither schizo-heterosexuality nor ego-dystonic heterosexuality has yet entered the literature. While perhaps Socarides cannot be faulted for inconsistency, since he views homosexuality as necessarily pathological, the APA's nomenclature seems odd to many clinicians in light of the organization's 1973 declassification of homosexuality per se (see Bayer, 1981).

Again, it is our purpose neither to find the line between true homosexuality and true heterosexuality, nor to resolve the problem of psychiatric nosology (but see Stoller, 1975). Rather, it is to point up the peculiarly unscientific character of many of the discussions of the question, and to note the problematic nature of our cultural assumptions about sexual orientation.

Our culture does not let people rest content with simply engaging in sexual behavior. It requires that they conceptualize that behavior as reflecting a sexual orientation and, moreover, it grossly stigmatizes one of the two categories it supplies. Finally, the *concept* of sexual orientation itself is so impoverished, and begs so many important questions, that it cannot help but do violence to the diversity of human sexuality. It is partly for this reason that some of the psychological constructions described in this paper seem so strained. Doubtless some people are most usefully described as denying their homosexuality, or, perhaps more accurately, as using these constructions to deny that there is a homosexual component to their sexuality. But I think others are, however awkwardly, showing us that formulating useful "objective" categories of sexual and affectionate feelings and behavior is a much more difficult task than we have acknowledged.

REFERENCES

Bayer, R. (1981). *Homosexuality and American psychiatry: The politics of diagnosis.* New York: Basic.

Boswell, J. (1980). *Christianity, social tolerance, and homosexuality: Gay people in Western Europe from the beginning of the Christian Era to the Fourteenth Century.* Chicago: University of Chicago Press.

Cass, V. C. (1979). Homosexual identity formation: A theoretical model. *Journal of Homosexuality, 4,* 219-235.

Crew, L., & Norton, R. (1974). The homophobic imagination: An editorial. *College English, 36,* 272-290.

Crowley, M. (1968). *The boys in the band.* New York: Farrar, Straus, & Giroux.

D. E. (1982). Mortimer on the Affair. *The Dial, 3*(3), p. 22.

Davison, G. C. (1982). Politics, ethics, and therapy for homosexuality. *American Behavioral Scientist, 25,* 423-434. (Also in Paul et al. (1982), pp. 80-98.)

Davison, G. C. (1976). Homosexuality: The ethical challenge. *Journal of Consulting and Clincial Psychology, 44,* 157-162.

Faber, D. (1980). *The life of Lorena Hickok, E.R.'s friend.* New York: William Morrow.

Fenichel, O. (1945). *The psychoanalytic theory of neurosis.* New York: Norton.

Gay, P. (1978). *Freud, Jews and other Germans: Masters and victims in modernist culture.* Oxford: Oxford University Press.

Goffman, E. (1974). *Stigma: Notes on the management of spoiled identity.* New York: Aronson. (Orig. pub. 1963.)

Grunfeld, F. V. (1979). *Prophets without honour: A background to Freud, Kafka, Einstein and their world.* New York: Holt, Rinehart & Winston.

Hart, J., & Richardson, D. (1981). *The theory and practice of homosexuality.* London: Routledge & Kegan Paul.

Hencken, J. D. (1982). Homosexuality and psychoanalysis: Toward a mutual understanding. *American Behavioral Scientist, 25,* 435-468. (Also in Paul et al. (1982), pp. 121-147.)

Hocquenghem, G. (1978). *Homosexual desire.* London: Allison & Bushby. (Orig. pub. 1972.)

Hoffman, M. (1972). The male prostitute. *Sexual Behavior, 2,* 16-21.

Marmor, J. (Ed.) (1980). *Homosexual behavior: A modern reappraisal.* New York: Basic.

Masters, W. H., & Johnson, V. E. (1979). *Homosexuality in perspective.* Boston: Little, Brown.

Paul, W., Weinrich, J. D., Gonsiorek, J. C., & Hotvedt, M. E. (Eds.) (1982). *Homosexuality: Social, psychological, and biological issues.* Beverly Hills: Sage.

Plummer, K. (1975). *Sexual stigma: An interactionist account.* London: Routledge & Kegan Paul.

Rechy, J. (1967). *Numbers.* New York: Grove.

Shapiro, D. (1965). *Neurotic styles.* New York: Basic.

Socarides, C. W. (1978). *Homosexuality.* New York: Aronson.

Stoller, R. J. (1975). *Perversion: The erotic form of hatred.* New York: Pantheon.

Sullivan, H. S. (1947). *Conceptions of modern psychiatry.* New York: William Alanson White Foundation.

Szasz, T. S. (1961). *The myth of mental illness.* New York: Dell.

Tripp, C. A. (1975). *The homosexual matrix.* New York: McGraw-Hill.

Waugh, E. (1945). *Brideshead revisited.* Boston: Little, Brown.

Biological Research on Homosexuality: Ansell's Cow or Occam's Razor?

Wendell Ricketts, MA (cand.)

San Francisco State University

"The cow is there," said Ansell, lighting a match and holding it over the carpet. No one spoke. He waited till the end of the match fell off. Then he said again, "She is there, the cow. There, now."

"You have not proved it," said a voice.

"I have proved it to myself."

"I have proved it to myself that she isn't," said the voice. "The cow is *not* there." Ansell frowned and lit another match.

"She's there for me," he declared. "I don't care whether she's there for you or not. Whether I'm in Cambridge or Iceland or dead, the cow will be there."

It was philosophy. They were discussing the existence of objects. Do they exist only when there is someone to look at them? Or have they a real existence of their own?

* * *

"Look here, Ansell. I'm there—in the meadow—the cow's there. You're there—the cow's there. Do you agree so far?"

"Well?"

"Well, if you go, the cow stays; but if I go, the cow goes. Then what happens if you stay and I go?"

E. M. Forster
The Longest Journey

ABSTRACT. Research based on the assumption that homosexuality can be traced to heredity, prenatal brain differentiation, or effects of gonadotropins in adulthood is reviewed. From a biological standpoint the studies are deficient in several respects: More or less accurate methods of hormone assay, uncertainty over the process of brain sexual differentiation in humans, lack of agreement regarding the role of various gonadotropins in human behavior, small samples, and lack of controls. Moreover, the biological research is based on unwarranted assumptions about human sexuality, sex differences, and sexual orientation that have been imported

---

The author obtained his Bachelor's degree in human sexuality, and is presently a graduate student at San Francisco State University. Requests for reprints should be addressed to the author, 1302 Sanchez, San Francisco, CA 94131.

65

from the social sciences and popular beliefs. The article questions why a biological basis for sexual orientation is expected, why biologists try to explain homosexuality but not heterosexuality, and what biologists mean by "homosexual." The author concludes that the biological research on homosexuality shows the ineluctable taint on "objective" science of personal beliefs and cultural prejudices.

A biological approach to the phenomenon of human homosexuality is not new. Biology has, in fact, made significant contributions to the notion of the immutable homosexual identity by attempting to root it deeply within the subcortical recesses or to attribute it to mysterious combinations of chromosomes. But homosexuality has not always been the intransigent personal identity it is widely believed to be today. Many sexual historians believe that the shift in social and scientific thinking about homosexuality, on behalf of which biology was pressed into service, began only in the nineteenth century.[1] Foucault (1978), for example, describes the transmutation of the homosexual:

> The nineteenth-century homosexual became a personage, a past, a case history, and a childhood, in addition to being a type of life, a life form, and a morphology, with an indiscreet anatomy and possibly a mysterious physiology. Nothing that went into this total composition was unaffected by his sexuality . . . . It was consubstantial with him, less as a habitual sin than as a singular nature . . . . Homosexuality appeared as one of the forms of sexuality when it was transformed from the practice of sodomy into a kind of interior androgyny, a hermaphroditism of the soul. The sodomite had been a temporary aberration; the homosexual was now a species. (p. 43)

One of the major nineteenth-century spokesmen for the idea of a personal homosexual identity was Karl Heinrich Ulrichs. Between 1864 and 1879 Ulrichs published his *Forschungen über das Rätsel der mannmännlichen Liebe* ("Researches on the Riddle of Love Between Men"), in which he put forth in estimable detail his theory of the "Third Sex." Hubert Kennedy, in his study of Ulrichs (1980/81), notes:

> Ulrichs found the basis for his theory in contemporary studies of embryology. He was particularly impressed with the fact that the future sexual organs are not differentiated in the early developmental stages of the human embryo . . . . This fact suggested to Ulrichs the possibility that an embryo could develop in either direction, both with regard to the differentiation of the sexual organs and to the sex drive . . . . Citing cases of known physical hermaphrodites, Ulrichs pointed out that, just as nature's "rule" is not always fol-

lowed in the differentiation of the sexual organs, so too the differentiation of the sex drive may vary from the usual rule. (p. 105)

The remarkable complexity of Ulrichs' classificatory scheme helped to relegate its details to the dusty halls of history, but not so with his rather rapturous expression of the special nature of the Third Sex: *anima muliebris virili corpore inclusa* (a female soul confined within a male body); indeed, Ulrichs noted:

The phrase "anima muliebris virili corpore inclusa" stands like a pillar of justice and the fangs of time will not come to gnaw it away. (*Memnon*, p. 15)[2]

Sigmund Freud knew Ulrichs' work and referred to the *anima muliebris* in his *Three Essays on the Theory of Sexuality* (1905/1975, p. 8). Freud, however, no less a product of his training as a neuroanatomist than of his Viennese culture, translated the word *anima* (soul) as *Gehirn* (brain) (1905/1961, p. 43). Although Freud rejected the notion of a "female brain," he entered into the dialogue among scientists of his day regarding the existence in the adult human brain of "sex centers" and of vestigial yet active elements of the "subordinated" embryonic sex (1905/1975, p. 9, n. 1).

Ulrichs was not blind to the good a biological theory could do for homosexuals threatened with arrest under Prussian sodomy laws. His theories allowed him to argue for leniency on the part of a friend caught *in flagrente* with a boy in a Mannheim park. An inborn (*angeboren*) homosexuality, Ulrichs knew, precluded the possibility of criminally prosecuting the homosexual who was, after all, guiltless in obeying the implacable call of nature.

If the political uses of a biological theory of homosexuality were first recognized by Ulrichs, they have been eagerly capitalized upon by modern "gay liberationists." More satisfying from the point of view that all guilty parties in the typical psychological/psychoanalytic paradigm of homosexuality are exonerated by biology—including not only the passive father, seductive mother, and constitutionally weak individual, but also child "molesters," homosexual teachers, and women with vagina dentata—the theory of inborn homosexuality also allows homosexuals to take their place beside blacks and women as a bona fide minority (see De Cecco & Shively, Note 1).

The popularity of theories of an innate homosexuality was boosted by the appearance in 1981 of Bell, Weinberg, and Hammersmith's *Sexual Preference.* After performing an elaborate, not to say byzantine, path analysis on retrospective data from 979 more or less homosexual men and women concerning their relationships with friends, parents, and siblings

from child- to adulthood; gender nonconformity; dating and sexual experiences; possible homosexual seductions and so forth, Bell et al. were
unable to support a social learning or psychoanalytic model of homosexuality. The final chapter in their book, entitled "Biology?", contains
this modest disclaimer:

> As much as we might wish it were otherwise, our own study does
> not include the kinds of data that would allow us to determine more
> precisely the extent to which biological history and constitution may
> contribute to sexual preference in adulthood. Nonetheless, *our find-
> ings are not inconsistent with what one would expect to find if, in-
> deed, there were a biological basis for sexual preference.* That is,
> our study provides no basis for rejecting biological explanations out-
> right. (p. 216; their emphasis)

Although Bell and his associates were rather circumspect in their conclusions about the role of biology in the etiology of homosexuality, they
managed to offend some biologists who, although they may have believed
in the futility of absolutist nature vs. nurture arguments, were less ready
to abandon the traditional territorial hostility between themselves and
social scientists. Likewise, sociologists and psychologists felt a certain
pang of jealousy as biology was seduced and social science somewhat
abandoned.

Sexual Preference was, however, welcomed by homosexual apolo-
gists, and the misinterpretations to which it has been subject are aptly
demonstrated by a fatuous review entitled "Born Gay" in the gay
magazine, *Christopher Street* (Herron, 1981). Gay politicoes, blissfully
unaware that some biologists have studied homosexuality precisely so
they could figure out how to prevent it, embraced Bell, Weinberg, and
Hammersmith's conclusion as the long-awaited exorcism of the demons
of Freudian and Bieberian psychology.

Within the field of biology itself, research and theory regarding the
genesis of human homosexuality has fallen into two major categories:
hormonal and genetic. Each of these areas of conjecture and research will
be dealt with separately and in more detail. Before I turn to these studies,
however, it is important to review the findings of animal research and to
understand the model animal behavior has provided for studying human
homosexuality.

THE ANIMAL MODEL

The animal species whose sexual behavior is commonly studied in the
laboratory exhibit mating behavior that is unmistakably sexually dimorphic. Sexually dimorphic behavior may be most simply expressed as be-

havior for which both sexes have the capacity but which is highly characteristic of one and not the other. Sexually dimorphic behavior varies greatly among animal species, and I will not attempt a description here (see Dewsbury, 1979, for a thorough overview). Researchers have devoted a great deal of attention to studying the effects of various gonadotropins on sexually dimorphic copulatory behavior in nonhuman mammals, chiefly rats, and have reliably documented the interchangeability of male and female mating behaviors under the right experimental conditions.[3] Noble (1979) concludes that sexual dimorphism in copulatory activity of rodents is "mainly differences in the amount of hormonal or external stimulation required to elicit the behavior rather than inherent differences in the capacity to execute the copulatory behaviors of the opposite sex" (p. 293).

In general it can be said that male and female mating behaviors, at least with respect to rats, consist of characteristic, quantifiable patterns of motor activity that occur within a relatively simple stimulus-response paradigm. This behavior is referred to as "lordosis" in the female rodent (or as "presenting" in female primates and other higher mammals) and as "mounting" in the male.

Dewsbury (1979) describes this behavior in some detail, pointing out that mating behavior in the adult male rat comprises mounting, thrusting, a series of intromissions, and a final ejaculation as well as genital grooming, ultrasonic vocalizations, and other behaviors (p. 5). He also notes the variety of proceptive behaviors in the female rat (p. 15).

The relevant research on the rat has explored the role of gonadal hormones in enhancing or extinguishing sexually dimorphic mating behaviors. Hormones may have an effect both during the critical period of sex differentiation when hypothalamic-pituitary organization takes place and in adulthood. Beach (1979) summarizes:

> The conventional working hypothesis is that during a "critical period" of organogenesis and embryonic differentiation, endogenously produced testosterone exerts "masculinizing" effects on the functional organization of CNS mechanisms designed to mediate male behaviour in adult life. If androgen is absent during the critical period, "masculine" mechanisms do not differentiate completely, but the alternate mechanisms associated with female behavior do become organized. This of course describes the normal course of events in the development of the female (p. 118) . . . . In terms of behavioural analysis the primary effect of testosterone on mating in adult rats can be expressed as follows T $\uparrow$ Pr $\female$ S$\rightarrow$ $\male$ R, or testosterone increases the probability that the feminine stimulus pattern will elicit the masculine response pattern. The analogous formula for oestrogen would be: 0 $\uparrow$ Pro$\male$S$\rightarrow$ $\female$ R. (p. 119)

This direct stimulus-response characteristic is less well defined in higher animals, and in primates "the effects of gonadal hormones on sexual activity are more permissive than obligatory, and this opens up the possibility for modulation of sexual behavior by other determinants, including learning" (Beach, 1979, p. 127). Ehrhardt and Meyer-Bahlburg (1981, p. 1316) cite the research of Goldfoot and Wallen as evidence that primate mating can be "profoundly" affected by social learning in childhood.[4]

With regard to homosexual behavior, Günter Dörner and his associates have been most prodigious in their efforts to provide a "rat model" for human homosexuality. In his early experiments, Dörner treated female rats with androgens during their perinatal hypothalamic organization period and again at puberty during their hypothalamic activation period. These animals showed no difference in mounting, an ejaculation-like pattern, and refractory latencies from untreated males (Dörner, 1968, p. 164). Dörner also noted that castration at birth with later estrogen substitution, although it produced female sexual behavior in genetic male rats, could not provide a model for human homosexuality because homosexual men were presumed to have normal androgen levels after puberty. When he succeeded in establishing homosexual behavior in neonatally castrated male rats later treated with androgens, Dörner felt he had found the model he sought. His hypothesis was that the initial deficiency of androgens during the critical period (which in humans is prenatal, not perinatal as in rats) led to the female differentiation of the hypothalamic "mating centre(s)." These centers later responded to increased testosterone levels in puberty with a "sex-unspecific activation leading to genuine homosexuality in a geno- and phenotypically male organism" (Dörner & Hinz, 1968, p. 387-388). Similarly, an androgenic excess during the critical period caused the differentiation of a male hypothalamus and, consequently, female homosexuality (Dörner, 1968).

Dörner further reported that a positive estrogen feedback effect (Hohlweg effect) could be demonstrated in response to LH injection in neonatally castrated male rats (Dörner, 1974). This effect, typical of normal females, was evidence of a hypothalamus with a cyclic—that is, female—organization. Because Dörner believed that a predominantly female-differentiated hypothalamus was the necessary substrate upon which testosterone was to act in adulthood to produce homosexual behavior in genetic males, he was convinced he had provided a complete explanation for the genesis of homosexuality. By 1975 he felt able to apply this model confidently to humans (Dörner, Rohde, Stahl, Krell, & Masius, 1975).

Although Dörner proposed the feminization of the male brain and masculinization of the female brain as mechanisms for the creation of male and female homosexuality respectively, he was at first silent on the question of what conditions led to the hormone anomalies his model implied. Two British researchers, MacCulloch and Waddington (1981; MacCulloch, 1980), provided possible missing links.

Regarding female homosexuals, MacCulloch and Waddington (1981) hypothesized that masculinization of the female brain came about not as a direct result of androgen excess, but because of progesterone shortage. Relying on evidence from experiments on guinea pigs, the two researchers concluded that progesterone functions both to feminize the female brain and to protect it from the androgenic effects of aromatized estrogens. Thus, in the absence of progesterone and in the presence of normal or elevated amounts of androgens and estrogens, "a genetically female brain would be differentiated as functionally male, with subsequent homosexual behavior (choice of female object)" (p. 343).

Experiments with rabbits, on the other hand, demonstrated that an immune reaction to testosterone in pregnant females could be passed through the placenta to male fetuses in the form of antibodies to testosterone. These genetic males would be born with a female reproductive system and with elevated testosterone levels. Excited by Brodie, Gartrell, Doering, and Rhue's (1974) finding of higher testosterone in homosexual men, MacCulloch and Waddington concluded that a similar autoimmune reaction to testosterone might be present in some women whose sons were homosexual.

HORMONE STUDIES OF HUMANS: ADULT HORMONE LEVELS

Biological models of human homosexuality have been informed most significantly by beliefs about the nature of maleness and femaleness, beliefs extrapolated largely from observations of nonprimate animals. The equation of homosexuality in men and women with the exhibition of opposite-sex, sexually dimorphic behaviors in animals compels the presumption that male homosexuals are men who are not quite masculine enough, that is, are failed men; and that female homosexuals are women who are not feminine enough.

Early experiments supported the notion that male homosexuals had androgen deficiencies. Glass, Deuel, and Wright (1940), for example, reported reduced androgens and elevated estrogens in their male homosexual subjects as compared to controls. A bit disconcerted by the overlap in values between their homosexual subjects and the heterosexual controls, Glass et al. had this to say: "Those few normal subjects [i.e. those with low androgen levels] may be latent homosexuals whereas the homosexuals with the high values may not be of the true constitutional type"

(p. 593). Glass et al. suggested that hormone assays could be helpful in diagnosing homosexuality and in distinguishing between "acquired, latent and congenital (constitutional) types" (p. 593).

As more was learned about the nature and function of the gonadotropins, which were first synthesized in the late 1920s, it became quite fashionable to treat homosexual men with large quantities of hormones, chiefly androgens. The idea, transparent as it was, was that virilizing hormones would restore both masculinity and that *sine qua non* of true manliness, heterosexuality.

Rosenzweig and Hoskins (1941), for example, reported on a case of a 46-year-old black male homosexual hospitalized with "constitutional psychopathic personality without psychosis" (p. 87). This patient, A. D., whom Rosenzweig and Hoskins considered "pronouncedly" homosexual, was also extremely effeminate: "[He] spends hours at his toilette [and with women] he talks as one woman to another" (p. 88). The patient apparently had one rather unladylike habit, however: He was preoccupied with defecation, "the significance of which is obvious in terms of psychoanalytic doctrine" (p. 88).[5] A.D. also had extremely large genitals, the only one of his features which Rosenzweig and Hoskins considered "masculine."

Nothing daunted, the doctors set about to cure A. D. of his effeminacy, his homosexuality, or both. From 16 October 1939 to 12 April 1940, A. D. received, for varying lengths of time, all of the following: oral doses of Stilbesterol; a subcutaneous testosterone implant; injections of gonadotropins from pregnant-mare serum, for which pituitary gonadotropic hormone was later substituted; dessicated thyroid to increase his receptivity to the other hormones; injections of testosterone propionate; emmenin, an estrogenic preparation; and estriol. A.D. experienced some nausea but the two doctors, who knew such things, decided it was not severe enough to discontinue the treatment. By the end of the experiment, however, Rosenzweig and Hoskins sadly had to conclude that "none of the drugs of the entire series gave rise to any detectable change in behavior" (p. 89). It was, they felt, a case "in which the homosexuality is of long-standing—35 years in this instance—and in which the personality structure has been altered at an early date [so that] the autogenous hormonal factors are no longer of significant potency" (p. 89).

For the most part, as it turns out, attempts to treat homosexuality with hormones were disappointing; far from turning male homosexuals into heterosexuals, administration of androgens often simply made them more sexually aroused (Gartrell, 1982; Glass & Johnson, 1944; Perloff, 1949).[6]

When Kinsey (1941) took issue with the Glass et al. paper (1940), he reported on the incidence of male homosexuality from what would eventually become *Sexual Behavior in the Human Male*. Kinsey insisted that any future research on the hormonal bases of homosexuality must take into account the fact that

> something between one fourth and one half of all males have demonstrated their capacity to respond to homosexual stimuli; that the picture is one of endless intergradation between every combination of homosexuality and heterosexuality; that it is impossible to distinguish so-called acquired, latent and congenital types; that there is every gradation between so-called actives and passives in a homosexual relation . . . . that both homosexual and heterosexual activities may occur coincidentally in a single period in the life of a single individual; that exclusive activities of any one type may be exchanged, in the brief span of a few days or a few weeks, for an exclusive pattern of the other type or into a combination pattern which embraces the two types . . . . that a large portion of the younger adolescents demonstrate the capacity to react to both homosexual and heterosexual stimuli; that there is a fair number of adults who show this same capacity; and that there is only a gradual development of the exclusive homosexual or exclusive heterosexual patterns which predominate among older adults. (p. 428)

For all of which Glass and Johnson thanked Dr. Kinsey kindly but demurred: "[I]f intergradation were to be thought of as vitiating classification the medical sciences would require revolution" (1944, p. 542). And so they would indeed.

Although conflicting reports may be found in the literature today regarding just what effect androgens do have on sexual behavior (Bancroft, 1978; Pirke, 1974; Rose, 1978), no one appears to believe that hormones administered in adulthood can affect the *direction* of the sexual drive. This has not stopped scientists from searching for adult endocrine correlates of homosexuality, however, and that literature is fairly extensive.

In 1971, Kolodny, Masters, Hendryx, and Toro published an investigation of testosterone levels in homosexual men. This was followed by a brief paper on the same group of men whose LH, FSH, and prolactin levels were then reported (Kolodny, Jacobs, Masters, Toro, & Daughaday, 1972). Having divided their subjects into subgroups on the basis of their Kinsey scale ratings, Kolodny et al. (1971) looked for a pattern of decreasing testosterone levels as subjects moved from less to greater homosexual activity; this they found, although the only significant differences were between the predominantly homosexual group (Kinsey 5s and 6s) and the heterosexual controls.

Kolodny and his associates have been soundly drubbed subsequently for their poor methodology (e.g., Gartrell, 1982; Meyer-Bahlburg, 1977). A number of their homosexual subjects were chronic marihuana smokers, which is now known to reduce testosterone levels (Kolodny, Masters, Kolodner & Toro, 1974); and four were azoospermic, a condition that suggests testicular disease. These factors may explain why only one other study (Starka, Sipova, & Hynie, 1975) has been able to duplicate the finding of Kolodny et al. (1971) of reduced testosterone levels in homosexual men. Nonetheless, their study is mentioned in the literature review of nearly every research article since, almost invariably without qualification. If Kolodny et al. cannot be credited with doing good research, they can at least be noted for ushering in a decade of interest in (dare I say clamor over) hormones and homosexuality.

Recent studies have focused primarily on total testosterone levels in men and women, but several have measured other hormones (see Birke, 1981, for a review). The two studies that found decreased total plasma testosterone in men have already been mentioned. Twelve studies found no significant differences between male homosexuals and heterosexuals (or between homosexuals and normal values): Barlow, Abel, Blanchard, and Mavissakalian (1974); Birk, Williams, Chasin, and Rose (1973); Doerr, Kockott, Bogt, Pirke, and Dittmar (1973); Dörner et al. (1975); Friedman, Dyenfurth, Linkie, Tendler, and Fleiss (1977); Jaffee, McCormack, and Vaitukaitis (1980); Livingstone, Sagel, Distiller, Morley, and Katz (1978); Parks, Korth-Schutz, Penny, Hilding, Dumars, Frasier, and New (1974); Pillard, Rose, and Sherwood (1974); Rohde, Stahl, and Dörner (1977); Stahl, Dörner, Ahrens, and Graudenz (1976); Tourney, Petrilli, and Hatfield (1975).

Two studies showed elevated free testosterone in males. The first was Brodie et al. (1974), where differences reached the level of significance. Birk et al. (1973) found no significant correlations between Kinsey scale rating and testosterone level for their 19 homosexual subjects, but the elevated testosterone levels in the sample, although within uppermost normal limits, were quite striking.

The three studies that measured the biologically active, *unbound* portion of testosterone report contradictory results. Rohde et al. (1977) and Stahl et al. (1976) showed significantly lower free testosterone in homosexuals, while Doerr, Pirke, Kockott, and Dittmar (1976) reported significantly higher mean free testosterone levels for homosexual subjects.

Regarding female homosexuality, Griffiths, Merry, Browning, Eisinger, Huntsman, Lord, Polani, Tanner, and Whitehouse (1974) assessed a number of urinary hormone metabolites; they found that 10 of their 42 homosexual subjects had elevated urinary testosterone and epitestosterone. Griffiths et al. used no control group and do not report individual values, although they say "some of the values were very much in excess of the normal range for females" (p. 554); the mean testosterone for the entire group, however, was well within normal limits. Only a few of their

42 subjects showed unusual values for any of the other hormones measured. Two subjects with unusual hormone levels were both taking oral contraceptives. In an early report on the same sample of women, Eisinger, Huntsman, Lord, Merry, Polani, Tanner, Whitehouse, and Griffiths (1972) admitted that "[H]ormonal concentrations in the 24 urine samples were well within the normal range, with allowances being made for any volunteers taking hormones" (p. 106).

Griffiths et al. were nonetheless suspicious of their results, and for quite other reasons. Having classified their subjects on the basis of whether they were the "active" (male) or "passive" (female) partner in homosexual relations, they made this comment regarding the discrepant testosterone values:

> Had the 10 subjects all been the "male" of the partnership the temptation to draw stronger conclusions would have been greater. However, this was not so, and in any case there was (not surprisingly) a marked preponderance of the "male" partners in the group of volunteers. (p. 554)

Gartrell, Loriaux, and Chase (1977) found significantly higher testosterone levels in a group of homosexual women; these are apparently the only studies of hormone levels in adult female homosexuals within the decade covered by this paper.[7]

Since these studies reflect a decade's worth of biological thinking about adult hormone levels and homosexuality, it is well to attend with some care to the particulars of their methodology. To begin with, the vast majority of studies of plasma hormones involved only one blood sample. Single-sample measures of hormones are notoriously suspect, due to secretion of hormones episodically or according to circadian or diurnal rhythms (Meyer-Bahlburg, 1977). Parks et al. (1974) measured LH, FSH, and testosterone in 12 adolescents (ages 16–19) and found major variations that would have made it difficult "to properly evaluate the hormonal status of a subject from only one hormone determination" (p. 800).

Nieschlag (1979) reports that testosterone flows from the testes in "short, secretory spikes, 6–7 usually occurring during the day" (p. 185). LH and FSH, being dependent upon a hypothalamic-pituitary-gonadal feedback system, are also likely to be affected by variations in testosterone. Nieschlag further points out that testosterone is suppressed by psychological stress (see also Kreuz, Rose, and Jennings, 1972), and by physical stress and exercise of long (but not short) duration (p. 189). The findings of Rohde et al. (1977) and Stahl et al. (1976) vis-à-vis decreased *free* testosterone in homosexuals, and of Stahl et al. (1976) of increased testosterone binding globulin (TeBG) in homosexuals, may be explained by the fact that the percentage of testosterone binding increases with age so that the free fraction decreases (Nieschlag, 1979). Indeed, the subjects in those two studies ranged from 20–49 (n = 50 Hs) and from 20–45 (n=78 Cs) in Rohde et al. and from 20–40 (n=35 Hs, 38Cs) in Stahl et al. In contrast, Doerr et al. (1976) found significantly higher free testosterone in his younger homosexuals than in controls (each group n=26, age 20–33).

Another major problem with a number of hormone studies is the lack of proper control groups. Several researchers used no controls at all (e.g., Barlow et al., 1974; Birk et al., 1973; Griffiths et al., 1974); several coopted controls from other studies going on in their laboratories (e.g., Brodie et al., 1974; Evans, 1972). Occasionally, homosexuals were matched with blatantly inappropriate controls; Pillard et al. (1974), for instance, compared volunteers from homophile organizations with soldiers in an officers training school who had been recruited for another study. Gartrell (1982), in her critique, points out these additional problems: The studies vary greatly "in the extent to which they controlled factors which are known to affect hormone measurements" (p. 175); the diversity of techniques of hormone measurement makes comparison across studies "difficult" (p. 178; see also Meyer-Bahlburg, 1977).

But more frustrating than any of this is the utter gravity with which investigators have contemplated any statistically significant finding. In medical research, as elsewhere, correlations must occasionally be due to chance or error; they seem particularly likely to be in the research so far reported, in which samples are so frequently small and differences between experimental and control groups so considerable. Some biological researchers appear to have forgotten that cardinal rule of statistical analysis: Correlation does not prove causality.

PRENATAL HORMONE CONDITIONS: APPLYING THE ANIMAL MODEL TO HUMANS

The belief that virilizing hormones are deficient in male but excessive in female homosexuals, or that feminizing hormones are elevated or reduced respectively, came from studies on many animal species in which sexually dimorphic behavior was demonstrated to depend directly on "activational" gonadotropins in puberty and adulthood. Similarly, speculations on inappropriately feminized or masculinized brains come from animal evidence supporting the view that such a brain is the substrate upon which hormones must act to create "homosexual" behavior in adults.

For perhaps obvious reasons, research on the effects of sex hormones during prenatal hypothalamic-pituitary-gonadal organization has not been conducted on humans. Most of what is believed to be true about sexual differentiation of the human brain, therefore, comes from animal experiments and from studies of individuals born with anomalies in prenatal sexual differentiation. In the case of such humans, prenatal hormone conditions are inferred from what can be observed about them in child- or adulthood.

The anomalies in sexual differentiation that are of interest here can be caused either by abnormalities in endogenous hormone manufacture or synthesis, such as congenital adrenal hyperplasia (adrenogenital syndrome) and testicular feminization (androgen insensitivity syndrome); or by exogenous conditions. (See reviews by Bancroft, 1978; Hines, 1982.)

In 1975 Dörner et al. reported research on the estrogen feedback response in homosexual men. Dörner et al. believed that an androgen deficiency in men during a critical hypothalamic organization period resulted in a feminized brain that would respond to the administration of estrogen with an increase in LH. Blood was drawn from 21 homosexual, 20 heteroseuxal, and 5 bisexual men, both before and after the men were injected with 20 mg Presomen (Premarin), an estrogen. Estrogen feedback, manifested as a primary drop in LH followed by a secondary rise above basal levels, was demonstrated in 13 of the homosexual men. Dörner et al. concluded that the occurrence of the response in homosexual men, along with the fact that the response was weaker than in "intact" women, was consistent with their theory of a predominantly female-differentiated brain in homosexual males.

Dörner, Geier, Ahrens, Krell, Münx, Sieler, Kittner, and Müller (1980) proposed a model for the mechanism by which the female-disposing androgen deficiency occurred in males. Studies of pregnant female rats had shown that exposure to stress produced an androgen deficiency in male rat fetuses and, subsequently, their feminization. Dörner et al. studied 865 homosexual males registered by venereologists in East Germany. They found that the relative frequency of homosexual births was significantly higher between 1940 and 1945, a World War II period during which Dörner et al. believed pregnant women had been exposed to the deleterious effects of stress. Dörner et al. Also mentioned "paternal deficiency" (father absence) and malnutrition as postnatal contributors to the higher proportion of homosexuals born during the war years. Aside from the rather gross generalizations about the effects of war on hundreds of thousands of women and children, the hypothesis of Dörner et al. puts them at the mercy of what Sigusch, Schorsch, Dannecker, and Schmidt (1982) call a "crude sociobiologism." It is so far as I know Dörner's only appeal to other than strictly biological factors to support his hypotheses.

Gadpaille (1980) noted Dörner's work on estrogen feedback in men and stated that "comparable but opposite findings have been reported in women with homosexual behavior" (p. 8). In point of fact, the study to which Gadpaille refers (Dörner, Rohde, Seidel, Haas, & Schott, 1976) was an investigation of the estrogen feedback response not in homosexual women, but in six male-to-female and four female-to-male pre-operative transsexuals. Dörner et al. do refer to "homosexual behavior" in these individuals, by which one presumes they mean, for example, physical sexual activity between a genetic female who believes she is not a female and a genetic female who believes she is.

Although Dörner et al. are irritating in their insistence on anchoring sexual orientation exclusively within the biologic unit, excluding the interpersonal and cognitive aspects of biological sex and sexual identity (cf. De Cecco & Ricketts, 1982), their conceptual rigidity is not surprising. Dörner et al. see transsexualism as an extreme variety of homosexuality (or perhaps homosexuality as a muted form of transsexualism):

> In view of the findings [that] increased androgen or oestrogen levels during different periods of sex-specific brain differentiation . . . may lead to female homosexuality or bisexuality . . . such a neuroendocrine-conditioned predisposition to female homo- or bisexuality in women may predispose again to the development of transsexualism. (pp. 24–25)

Unfortunately, there are major difficulties with both studies. First, in Dörner et al. (1975), the Hohlweg effect was not demonstrated in the bisexual men, who would have been expected to show a weaker estrogen feedback than the homosexuals but a stronger one than the heterosexuals. In fact, the LH response of bisexuals was more negative than that of the heterosexuals. Moreover, seven of the 20 heterosexual men *did* show the response by the 96-hour point.[8] Second, Dörner's et al. (1976) insistence on conflating homosexuality and transsexualism is more willful than theoretically or empirically sound; under such circumstances serious consideration of this work is difficult. Finally, Kulin and Reiter (1976) demonstrated that estrogen feedback can be present in normal adult men. The effect may be blocked by testosterone and is apparently maturational; that is, it does not appear until late in, or after, puberty.

More damaging evidence against Dörner's hypothesis of a female-differentiated brain in male homosexuals comes from studies of the estrogen feedback effect in XY males with the testicular feminization syndrome, individuals whose levels of circulating testosterone are normal but who, because of a genetic defect, lack the specific protein receptors required to utilize testosterone at the target cell level. In two studies (Aono, Miyake, Kinusaga, Kurachi, & Matsumoto, 1978; VanLook, Hunter, Corker, & Baird, 1977), genetic males with testicular feminization were tested; none of the seven subjects in the two samples showed the Hohlweg effect typical of some male homosexuals in the 1975 study of Dörner et al.

Testicular feminized males, in whom androgen deprivation during fetal life is demonstrable rather than hypothetical as in homosexual males, would be expected to show a dramatic estrogen feedback response. Admittedly, it is not clear whether neural tissue in testicular feminized males is as unresponsive to androgens as is gonadal and other peripheral tissue; nonetheless, Dörner's own argument is that sexual differentiation of human hypothalamic tissue is controlled by levels of circulating gonadotropins during critical periods. If so, it is surprising that studies of the closest human approximation of his androgen-deprived male rats should fail to support this important link in the model.

Other work has been done on the sexual behavior of testicular feminized males. Masica, Money, and Ehrhardt (1971) reported on 10 TF patients followed up in late adolescence or early adulthood. Of the eight patients who had experienced sexual activity with another person, none had had homosexual relationships or erotic fantasies. Money and Ogunro (1974) reported on another 10 patients with partial androgen insensitivity (Reifenstein's syndrome). Of the two patients raised as girls, one was exclusively heterosexual in dreams and sexual activity, and the other had had a single homosexual experience. Seven of the eight patients reared as males had had only heterosexual experience and heterosexual erotic dreams and fantasies. The eighth reported no sexual activity with anyone.

Follow-up studies of genetic females with congenital adrenal hyperplasia have been somewhat more extensive. In CAH, a genetic defect of the adrenal cortices results in an inability to synthesize cortisone from androgen; instead, the hyperfunction of the adrenal cortex causes a surplus of androgen that masculinizes the genitalia of genetic females. If it is presumed that prenatal excess of androgen affects differentiation of the brain as well as of the genitalia, CAH women, particularly if they received cortisone treatment after a period of prolonged virilization, might be parallel to Dörner's (1968) androgenized female rats.

The research on CAH women, however, is far from conclusive. Ehrhardt, Evers, and Money (1968) reported on 23 CAH females from 21–63 years old at the time of follow-up. Of the 17 who had had sexual experiences with another person, 12 had engaged in heterosexual relationships exclusively, three (possibly four) had had homosexual as well as heterosexual relationships, and one provided no information. Of the 12 who were exclusively heterosexual in physical sexual activity, five had had erotic homosexual dreams or fantasies and seven had not.

Lev-Ran (1974), on the other hand, reported on 18 patients with late-treated CAH, not one of whom had experienced homosexual erotic fantasies, dreams or sexual activity. Since her study was conducted in the USSR, one might conclude that the single factor capable of overriding the putative effects of fetal masculinization on female sexual behavior is Soviet communism.

Money and Schwartz (1977) reported on 17 CAH patients 16-25 years old at follow up. Of eight patients who had engaged in physical sexual activity with a partner, five had had only partners of the opposite sex and three had had some degree of homosexual involvement; only one of these three had experienced exclusively homosexual activity. Six reported only heterosexual erotic dreams or fantasies, one reported only homosexual dreams and five reported both; data were missing for five others. Baker (1980) reported a follow-up of Ehrhardt, Epstein, and Money's (1968) sample of 15 early-treated CAH patients raised as girls:

> The general pattern of findings was that both interest in and experience with such heterosexual activities as dating, necking, petting and intercourse were delayed. Of the five girls who were not interested, four were the four youngest in the sample. The fifth was a 20-year-old socially-withdrawn girl who avoided close relationships with men and women. Only one woman reported homosexual fantasies or experiences. She had had both heterosexual and homosexual relationships. (p. 84)

The identification of heterosexual or homosexual physical sexual activity in CAH and TF patients is generally based upon sex of rearing. That is, a CAH female, although chromosomally XY, is usually considered to be heterosexual if she engages in physical sexual activities with another individual reared and socialized as a male. In a breathtaking display of conceptual prestidigitation, however, Money and Dalery (1976) reported on three CAH patients reared, with surgical correction, as boys. Although these individuals lived in adulthood as men, considered themselves to be men, were perceived by others as men, and were sexually attracted exclusively to adult women, Money and Dalery discerned a rather more complicated wrinkle in their case. The three patients, they thought, exemplified

> a formula for creating the perfect female homosexual—homosexual on the criteria of chromosomal and gonadal sex—[which] is to take a chromosomal and gonadal female fetus and to flood the system with a masculine hormone during the critical period when the external genitals and sexual pathways in the brain are being differentiated. Then assign the baby as a boy at birth and rear him unambiguously as a boy, making sure that hormonal puberty, at the appropriate age, is masculinizing.

With regard to exogenous hormones, Money and Mathews (1982) reported on 12 females born to mothers who had been treated in pregnancy with synthetic progesterone in the hope of preventing miscarriage. It was not known at the time that these progestins had androgenic effects as well; as a result, some offspring of the treated mothers were born with superficially masculinized genitalia. Psychosexual data were available for only six women, none of whom had had homosexual or "bisexual" erotic fantasies, dreams, or sexual experiences.

Yalom, Green, and Fisk (1973) conducted a more detailed study of 40 nondiabetic boys born to diabetic mothers treated in pregnancy with estrogen and progesterone to prevent miscarriage. Twenty 16- and 17-year-old boys were compared to 22 same-aged controls whose mothers were not treated in pregnancy. Subjects were evaluated on a battery of projective psychological tests; were interviewed extensively regarding participation in sports, interest and skill in mechanical and electrical activities, school subjects, future plans for college or military service, how close or far they were in the class hierarchy from the bully who could "beat everyone up," clothes and grooming, erotic fantasies, masturbation, physical sexual activity and so on; and were given a physical exam. Finally, each boy was led into an open field where he was "asked to catch a ball, field ground balls, swing a baseball bat, and run 30.5m while the experimenter, ostensibly timing his speed, observed his physical mannerisms" (p. 555).

This rather exhaustive series of tests was intended to reveal each subject's masculinity and degree of heterosexual development. Skill at baseball, having performed the evolutionary marvel of becoming a sex-linked male trait in less than 150 years, was of course considered evidence of normal masculine behavior. The trend was for the experimental boys to be less heterosexually developed and less masculine than the controls, although this was not a statistically significant finding. The representative description Yalom et al. (1973) give of one 16-year-old boy, Jim, who fell into the lower quartiles on masculinity and heterosexual development bears quoting in part:

> Jim performed the athletic tasks in a decidedly feminine manner. He threw the ball awkwardly and with little force . . . . He swung a bat through a very short arc with little force with elbows bent and with no breaking of the wrists. He ran mincingly with arms clasped near his chest. (p. 560)

The case of Jim is particularly remarkable because it is perhaps the first instance of a feminine boy being defined by wrists that were too stiff, not too limp.

In summing up these studies on prenatal sex hormone anomalies in humans, one must bear several points in mind. First, the degree of sensitivity of human neural tissue to sex hormones has not been conclusively demonstrated. Although tonicity or cyclicity of the CNS in rodents is directly dependent upon early exposure to gonadotropins, it is less clear in humans whether hormone conditions induce sexual differentiation of the hypothalamic-pituitary functions in so straightforward a manner (Hines, 1982, p. 58; MacLusky & Naftolin, 1981, p. 1295).

Second, it is impossible to determine the exact character of the anomalous prenatal hormone environment by studying adults with various kinds of endocrinopathies in sexual differentiation. Third, because individuals in homosexual relationships do not commonly suffer from genital abnormalities, sexual differentiation of the brain, if it is instrumental in the genesis of homosexuality, must occur after gonadal differentiation. But biologists can be little more certain than this regarding the timing of the "critical period" of CNS sensitivity. Moreover, cyclic (female) functions may be more susceptible to gonadotropins during different periods of fetal development than tonic (male) functions (MacLusky & Naftolin, 1981, p. 1296).

Finally, the practice of "accounting [for] the disorder [i.e., homosexuality] by use of the concept of a critical period cannot be accomplished without empirical demonstration of such a period" (Goy & McEwen, 1980, p. 72).

Studies of adults with CAH, TF, or exogenous hormone abnormalities cannot, in fine, be used to prove or disprove any theory of prenatal hormone influences on sexual orientation. The only conclusion we can draw at present regarding hypotheses of prenatal hormone influence on sexual orientation is that they are almost without exception untestable in humans. Nonetheless, prenatal hormone theories of homosexual etiology continue to be popular, even among researchers who consider the search for gonadotropin pathology in adult homosexuals an essentially fruitless endeavor. Perhaps part of the lure of prenatal theories lies in the fact that they cannot be conclusively disproved at present and that there is enough animal evidence to obfuscate the very real poverty of knowledge about the sexual differentiation of the human brain.

CONCLUSIONS

The research reviewed in this paper is predicated on the belief that there is some biological antecedent[9]—whether heredity, prenatal brain differentiation, or effects of gonadotropins in adulthood—of homosexuality. I have attempted up until now to evaluate the medical and biological research on its own grounds; that is, from the standpoint of biology. But I can do so only half-heartedly: more-or-less-accurate methods of hormone assay, uncertainty over the process of brain sexual differentiation in humans, lack of agreement regarding the role of various gonadotropins on human behavior, small samples, and lack of adequate controls—these difficulties from within the studies themselves are secondary in importance to the conceptual naivete and theoretical barrenness that characterize most of the biological research. In order to understand the contributions, as well as the unique failings, of biology, we must first rid ourselves of the belief that biological research is somehow more pure, more objective, more scientific than any other. And we must reject the idea that medico-biological research is immune to the influences of politics and personal prejudice. It is necessary to distinguish between the objectivity of *data* and the unquestionable subjectivity of the context in which research questions are asked in the first place. Moreover, when biologists turn to such matters as human homosexuality, they must rely on concepts from the social sciences, many of which translate rather poorly into biological terms. It seems quite clear, for example, that what some biologists call ''homosexuality'' in animals is a far stretch from what can be observed in humans. The assumptions about human sexuality, sex differences, and sexual orientation that doctors and biologists have made might be summed up in the following major points.

1) *Why ought we to expect there to be a biological basis for sexual orientation?* This may seem like a naive question, and I suppose it is, but it is one biologists must answer. The argument that homosexuality must have a biological basis simply because human beings are biological organisms is not particularly satisfying, falling, as it does, into the same self-serving category as the typical psychoanalytic response to criticisms of that field, e.g., ''If you don't recognize the effect of the unconscious on your behavior it's because it is unconscious.'' The fulcrum of a great deal of biological thought in this regard is, as Gadpaille (1980) put it, that the human brain is ''free to be uniquely human only with its shared mammalian heritage as its foundation'' (p. 17). It would be very unusual, of course, if human sexual behavior were unaffected by biological processes refined through eons of human evolution. Yet there is no reason to believe that human sexuality is the direct, immediate result of variations in hormones, of sexual differentiation of the brain or of genetic factors. If a simple link existed between human homosexuality and biology, it would undoubtedly have been found by now. Nonetheless, the effects of the *belief* in a cause-and-effect relationship between biology and homosexuality are significant.

With regard to animals, particularly rodents, on the other hand, gonadotropin levels do exert a direct influence on sexually dimorphic behavior. The question, of course, is whether this suggests a model for human behavior. In other words, is the hormonally demasculinized, lordotic male rat an analog of human homosexuality? Some biological researchers, it is clear, exercise little for caution in extrapolating directly from animal research to human behavior. Several points are relevant here.

In experiments, only the hormonally treated animal is considered homosexual. In other words, if an untreated male mounts a hormonally demasculinized male exhibiting lordosis, only the mounted rat is "homosexual." Likewise with female rats; only the mounting female is homosexual. (See Birke's, 1981, review; Dörner, 1968; Dörner & Hinz, 1968.) According to this model, then, only male homosexuals who receive penetration and only homosexual females who metaphorically, if not actually, penetrate other females are the "true" homosexuals. It scarcely needs to be said that this is a model based on reproduction, and that in the case of animal experiments the animal that deviates most strikingly from its "proper" reproductive role is the one considered homosexual. The penetration (i.e., symbolic insemination) of the mounted treated male by the untreated male and the act of reception (i.e., symbolic containment) by the untreated female at the mercy of a virilized amazon mouse—these are the "heterosexual" responses of normal animals behaving as appropriately as possible given the exigencies of the same sex situation.

Furthermore, because these behaviors (i.e., lordosis and mounting), if they are observed in the sex other than the one for which they are deemed appropriate, are themselves evidence of homosexuality, one is forced to the conclusion in human terms that all homosexuals may really be *bisexual*. According to the animal model, when a male inserts his penis he is behaving like a male and when he receives penetration, literally or figuratively, he is behaving like a female—regardless of the sex of his partner. This is a belief that has currency not only among some biologists but among prison inmates (Wooden & Parker, 1982, *passim*). In other words, homosexuals are made by opposite sex gender traits, an explanation that sounds unpleasantly familiar to anyone acquainted with the usual sociopsychological interpretations of homosexuality.

Biologists who subscribe to the animal model must on the one hand argue that a *type of behavior* is sexually dimorphic, regardless of the existence of a partner, or of the sex of the partner, if one is present. On the other hand, they must argue that the *choice of partner* is sexually dimorphic, which means that "normal" males must be biologically programed not only to mount and thrust but also to do so only with a female. Conceivably, then, anomalies can occur in the behavior mode, in the object mode, or both. Males could find themselves mounting and thrusting with admirable vigor, but with males instead of females. Alternatively, females might find themselves with a desire for male partners but with an irritating tendency to insist upon mounting them. Bisexuals could be those who mount, thrust, and lordose, but only with partners of the opposite sex; they could be those who pursue objects of both sexes but who, once they get them, rigidly insist on either mounting and thrusting or on lordosing, but not both; they could be individuals who mount, thrust, and lordose, and who do so with reckless disregard for the biological sex of their partners. Dörner and Hinz (1968), in spite of themselves, have helped to make clear the absurdity of animal models of homosexuality. In one experiment, demasculinized, lordotic male rats were caged with androgenized, aroused female rats. The "homosexual" females mounted the "homosexual" males with the result that each animal managed to behave both heterosexually (by the criterion of object choice) and homosexually (by the criterion of sexually dimorphic mating behavior) at exactly the same moment.

Because humans regularly "mount" and "lordose" independently of their partners' sex, and because humans can wind up doing so with one, the other, or both sexes, the animal model becomes utterly distorted. Object choice may be considered a sexually dimorphic behavior only if it is believed to be an aspect of, or the same as, gender identity (or gender identity/role, as Money, 1980, put it). This is what many biological researchers appear to have believed, and thus it should come as no real surprise that we find ourselves left with the familiar equation: male = masculine = heterosexual; female = feminine = heterosexual.

A number of researchers have, in fact, preoccupied themselves with attempting to figure out which homosexuals are "butch" or active and which are "femme" or passive, on the theory that nelly men and macho women are "more" homosexual. Griffiths' et al. (1974) comments regarding the "male" partners in lesbian relationships have already been mentioned; Starka et al. (1975) included in their sample 18 "feminine-disposed" male homosexuals and three with "virile reactions." Rohde's et al. (1977) and Dörner's (1979) reports reflect the long-time interest of the Dörner group in the differences between "effeminized" and "non-effeminized" male homosexuals and between "virilized" and "non-virilized" lesbians; in these studies, presumably, individuals who are homosexual and who depart from social sex role sterotypes represent an intermediate category between sex-role-conforming homosexuals, on the one hand, and transsexuals (see Dörner et al., 1976). Doerr et al. (1973, 1976) classified male homosexuals on the basis of whether they were "passive" insertees or "active" insertors. And Pillard et al. (1974) ascertained the femininity of their male homosexual subjects by asking them such questions as "Do friends ever refer to you with feminine names or pronouns?" But it was Perkins (1981) who appeared most overwhelmed by a certain Linnaean compulsion to create taxonomies of homosexuals. Her subjects fell into no less than seven categories based both on whether they exhibited "inverted" sexual behavior and on whether or not they considered themselves fully female in "psychosexual identity." One is hard-pressed, of course, to argue that some individuals involved in homosexual relationships do not depart from social sex role stereotypes; of course they do. On the other hand, heterosexual interest does not pre-

clude the adoption of certain, shall I say, bohemian sex role characteristics, and it is striking that researchers have so often ignored this fact.

2) *Why is it that biologists have felt compelled to explain only homosexuality?* I know of no attempts in the literature to explain how *heterosexuality* comes about as a result of prenatal brain organization; little interest
is apparent in a general theory of how sexual orientation develops under
the influence of biological factors. It is obvious that many researchers
have considered homosexuality *a priori* pathological and have attempted
to find out why from the standpoint of biology. A kind of heterosexual
chauvinism is thus coupled with the belief that homosexuals *ought* to be
different, and it is here that the influence of politics and cultural and personal prejudice comes to bear most strongly on the supposed objectivity
of biological research on sexual orientation.

Some researchers are unabashed in their desire to find ways to treat or
prevent homosexuality; Dörner has written for years about discovering a
hormonal "prophylaxis." Goy and McEwen (1980), in their review of
Dörner's research make this observation:

> Hence, according to Dörner, psychosexual orientation in humans
> may be based, at least in part, on discrepancies between the genetic
> sex and the sex-specific hormone level during brain development in
> prenatal life. Therefore, methods were developed for the determina-
> tion of genetic sex and sex-specific hormone levels in amniotic
> fluids in order to detect and possibly to correct such discrepancies in
> prenatal life. (p. 69)

Müller, Orthner, Roeder, König, Bosse, and Kloos (1974), as well as
Dieckmann and Hassler (1975), as other examples, have used stereotactic
hypothalamotomy (brain lesions) to treat "cases" of homosexuality because of the conviction, as the former state, that "abnormal sexual feelings are above all associated with a functionally defective hypothalamus"
(p. 103).

Can it be other than the most fascinating accident that researchers' conclusions regarding what is biologically normal sexuality coincide precisely with the last five or six hundred years of Western cultural prejudice
against homosexual behavior? Indeed, it should be pellucidly clear that it
is no accident and that such prejudice is what Sigusch et al. (1982) call the
"invisible employer" in most biological research on homosexuality.[10]

Geneticists have further confused the issue by proposing theories that
disregard their own caveats: Homosexuals do not arrive, preformed like
homunculi, through the action of a single gene or even combinations of a
few specific genes. A hereditary explanation implies expression of homosexuality via the unique physiology of a particular individual, but the
mechanisms by which genes transform themselves into living individuals

with homosexual behavior, fantasies, and relationships are left undefined by genetic explanations. Finally, although geneticists have spent decades arguing whether or not homosexuality runs in families, they seem to have learned little from the common knowledge that heterosexuality does.

3) What do biological researchers mean when they use the term "homosexual"? Often in biological research, as in sociological research where it is somehow less forgiveable, the sexual orientation of research subjects is simply not assessed. Participants may be presumed to be homosexual because they are recruited from what are quaintly referred to as "homophile" organizations. They may be asked if they are homosexual or an interviewer (frequently a psychiatrist) may decide for them. Sometimes they are assessed on the Kinsey scale which, with all its limitations, is perhaps better than nothing. The use of the Kinsey scale, however, usually means that sexual orientation is determined largely on the basis of physical sexual activity. Homosexual subjects may come from prisons or from psychiatric patient populations. Heterosexual subjects typically are laboratory workers (who couldn't possibly be homosexual), undefined groups of individuals, or controls drawn from other experiments in progress in the laboratory. Their sexual orientation is particularly unlikely to be assessed, which means that the extent of their homosexual experience is not known. Homosexual subjects in some studies report heterosexual sex, occasionally as much heterosexual sex as homosexual sex. A number of studies grouped homosexuals and transsexuals together (see Meyer-Bahlburg, 1977, for a review). It is only fair to say that some studies do exist in which controls were carefully matched with experimental subjects, and in which sexual orientation was a bit more reliably measured, but it is these that have most consistently failed to show differences between homosexuals and controls.

Researchers' apparent inability to obtain "pure" samples of heterosexuals and homosexuals, however, far from being an artifact, is a reflection of real life. Saliba's data (Note 2) demonstrate that an individual's choice of a self-label of bisexual, heterosexual, or homosexual can depend on any number of factors, among which the biological sex of one's partner is not always the most important. It is not surprisingly more difficult to find faithful adherents to either religion, particularly when erotic fantasy and love relationships are taken into consideration.

Notwithstanding this embarrassment of variation, most researchers have attempted to form, out of whatever unlikely clay they had in hand, an unsullied dichotomy comprising two and only two discrete categories, heterosexual and homosexual. This rigid compartition of heterosexuality and homosexuality runs throughout the genetic and hormonal literature, despite the fact that devising a neat biological theory of sexual orientation is a bit tricky when the dependent variable obstinately refuses to stand still and be measured. Consequently, although there is no reason why it should be impossible for biologists to discover some plausible connections between neuroendocrine conditions and sexual orientation, they are more likely to hear a thud where no apple fell.

Explanations of a direct cause-and-effect relationship between biological factors and sexual orientation falter because they cannot embrace the complexity and variety of human sexual behavior. Not only must they account for both exclusive heterosexuality and exclusive homosexuality, but they must also explain gradations of homosexuality and heterosexuality, bisexuality, exclusive sexual behavior with one sex coupled with fantasies about the other, and, indeed, the existence of fantasies themselves. Even if biologists were able to solve the mysteries of these combinations of components of sexual identity, they would not have accounted for a rather more complicated problem. The belief that the biological sex of one's partner is the single most important aspect of sexual relationships allows only a limited understanding of how men and women select partners; form alliances; fall in and out of love; integrate sexuality into their lives; and deal with perhaps conflicting needs for domination and submission, masculinity and femininity, autonomy and attachment, security and wanderlust.

Having set about to discover differences between heterosexuals and homosexuals, biologists have had no alternative but to conduct their research within the parameters of a particularly powerful but dubious presumption; *viz.,* the existence of heterosexual and homosexual personalities and identities. In this regard, modern sexual biologists show a certain conceptual loyalty to such nineteenth-century figures as Ulrichs, Hirschfeld, and von Krafft-Ebing. Under such a theory, the homosexual is identifiable chiefly by his or her distinct and remarkable biology, and only secondarily by the desire to have relationships with partners of the same sex.

Biologists in favor of hormonal theories have been forced to strip homosexual relationships of their social and emotional context in order to make them fit models created for nonhuman, largely nonprimate, animals. Geneticists, having reduced the area of conjecture to the submicroscopic level of genes, have moved even farther away from an appreciation of the complexity of the relationships implied by the labels "heterosexual" and "homosexual." Considering homosexuality a condition traceable, like albinism, in family histories has given it a certain substance, but has contributed little to an understanding of sexual identity.

For now the real question seems not to be whether human sexual identity is influenced primarily (or solely) by innate conditions as opposed to learning and environment, but whether it will be biologists or social scientists who prevail in demonstrating the conceptual barrenness of their theories, the arrogance of their research, and the ineluctable taint on "objective" science of personal beliefs and cultural prejudices.

At this point we are left with the unsatisfactory conclusion that we know too little about the human brain or the effects of hormones upon it, or about the contributions of heredity, to construct a parsimonious and viable biological theory of sexual orientation—an observation Freud made almost 70 years ago in the conclusion of his *Three Essays.*

What perhaps can be said now is that investigating the beliefs and biases of previous researchers and theorists is a valuable tool in forming the understanding necessary to grasp the mind-boggling complexity of human sexual relationships. I hope to have contributed something useful to that investigation.

NOTES

1. See Richardson, Diane. "The dilemma of essentiality in homosexual theory," *Journal of Homosexuality,* 1984, *9,* in press.

2. My translation.

3. See, for example, Michael, R. P., & Bonsall, R. W. (1979). Hormones and the sexual behavior of rhesus monkeys. In C. Beyer (Ed.), *Endocrine control of sexual behavior.* New York: Raven Press; Nobel, R. G. (1979). Male hamsters display female sexual responses. *Hormones and Behavior, 12,* 293-298; and Sachs, B. D. & Pollack, E. I. (1973). Sexual behavior: Normal male patterning in androgenized female rats. *Science, 181,* 770-772.

4. See Goldfoot, D. A., & Wallen, K. In D. J. Chivers, & J. Herbert (Eds.) (1978). *Recent advances in primatology. Volume I: Behaviour,* pp. 155-159. New York: Plenum Press.

5. The good doctors might well have been reminded, as Swift so eloquently pointed out, that even "Celia shits."

6. On the other side of the Atlantic, for reasons that are not quite clear to me, the opposite theory prevailed. Homosexual males were not unmanly and in need of an androgenic boost; they were hypersexual and in need of taming. Sand and Okkels (1938) reported on more than 100 repeat offenders (including homosexuals and others with "psychosexual aberrations") castrated by authority of the Danish Sterilization Act of 1 June 1929. They noted that

> the results of the castration have been very gratifying from a criminalistic point of view; the provisional report says that only a single individual, a homosexual, has been guilty of repeated offences. All the [others] state that the pathologically [sic] or excessive libido has completely disappeared. (p. 374).

Sand and Okkels concluded that the testes may not be the "only causal site of sexual abnormality" but that "in removing this link [i.e. the interstitial tissue of the testis] the final result (disturbances manifestative as hypersexualisme or homosexualisme) can be checked" (p. 374). The hypersexual theory did take hold in America as well (see Laughlin, 1914, for example), but the hormone deficiency theory seems to have been more popular.

7. Kenyon (1974) reviewed research on female homosexuality up until that time, including hormonal and genetic studies. See also Meyer-Bahlburg's (1979) review.

8. In Fall 1982, Richard Green and Brian Gladue (Long Island Research Institute, SUNY Stony Brook) began recruiting heterosexual and homosexual males, heterosexual females and male-to-female transsexuals for a large and more carefully controlled attempt to re-evaluate Dörner's estrogen feedback finding. (See Bohn, 1982.)

9. The biological search for the causes of homosexuality has extended beyond hormones and sexual differentiation of the brain to include the possibility of identifying an inherited factor. Because the mysteries of genes and chromosomes began to yield themselves up to scientists decades before the gonadotropins had been synthesized, some of the earliest speculations regarding links between biology and homosexuality centered around a potential genetic component. (See, for example, Krafft-Ebing, 1886/1950, on *erbliche Belastung,* hereditary taint, in "antipathic sexual interest," p. 349 *et passim.*

10. Ted Bohn (1982) in an article in the gay press, blasts biological research on homosexuality not only because he believes it is an attempt to wage "medical war" upon homosexuals, but because he feels scientists have a political and moral obligation not to investigate the causes of homosexuality in a "homophobic" society. Information from such studies, Bohn says, could be used to strengthen the "arsenal" or those who wish to eliminate homosexuality by medical means. Bohn also makes the point that recent arguments in favor of the acceptance of homosexuality have revolved around attempts to show that homosexuals are really the same as heterosexuals. Bohn feels that heterosexuals and homosexuals are fundamentally different, but calls for a "healthy affirmation" of these differences rather than discrimination on account of them. It does seem to be true that differences between heterosexuals and homosexuals, when they are found in biological research, tend to be interpreted to the disadvantage of the homosexuals. On the other hand, the research on differences among the sexual orientations also affirms the heterosexual and homosexual identities in which Bohn apparently believes. In that regard, Bohn probably has more in common with Dörner than either of them would care to say. Nonetheless, the insistence on the heterosexual/homosexual dichotomy is largely cant, both for social and natural scientists and for gay liberationists. No one knows exactly why heterosexuals and homosexuals ought to be different, and the blatant tautology of the hypotheses appears to have escaped careful attention: Heterosexuals and homosexuals are considered different because they can be divided into two groups on the basis of the belief that they can be divided into two groups.

REFERENCE NOTES

1. De Cecco, J. P., & Shively, M. S. (in press). *The heterosexual and homosexual identities: The normalization of sexual relationships.*
2. Saliba. P. (1983). *Variability in sexual orientation.* Manuscript submitted for publication.

REFERENCES

Aono, T., Miyake, A., Kinusaga, T., Kurachi, T., & Matsumoto, M. (1978). Absence of positive feedback effect of oestrogen on LH release in patients with testicular feminization syndrome. *Acta Endocrinologica, 87,* 259-267.

Baker, S. W. (1980). Biological influences on human sex and gender. *Signs, 6*(1), 80-96.

Bancroft, J. (1978). The relationship between hormones and sexual behaviour in humans. In J. B. Hutchinson (Ed.), *Biological determinants of sexual behaviour.* New York: John Wiley.

Barlow, D. H., Abel, G. G., Blanchard, E. B., & Mavissakalian, M. (1974). Plasma testosterone levels and male homosexuality: A failure to replicate. *Archives of Sexual Behavior, 3*(6), 571—575.

Beach, F. A. (1979). Animal models for human sexuality. In *Sex, hormones and behaviour.* Ciba Foundation Symposium, *62.* Amsterdam: Excerpta Medica.

Bell, A. P., Weinberg, M. S., & Hammersmith, S. K. (1981). *Sexual preference: Its development in men and women.* Bloomington: Indiana University Press.

Birk, L., Williams, G. H., Chasin, M., & Rose, L. I. (1973). Serum testosterone levels in homosexual men. *New England Journal of Medicine, 289*(23), 1236-1238.

Birke, L. (1981). Is homosexuality hormonally determined? *Journal of Homosexuality, 6*(4), 35-49.

Bohn, T. (1982, November 17). The politics of research on homosexuality: Controversial SUNY Stony Brook hormone research. *Long Island Connection,* pp. 12-14, 25.

Brodie, H. K. H., Gartrell, N., Doering, C., & Rhue, T. (1974). Plasma testosterone levels in heterosexual and homosexual men. *American Journal of Psychiatry, 131*(1), 82-83.

De Cecco, J. P., & Ricketts, W. (1982). Physical changing of gender. *Medical Aspects of Human Sexuality, 16*(7), 97.

Dewsbury, D. A. (1979). Description of sexual behavior in research on hormone-behavior interactions. In C. Beyer (Ed.), *Endocrine control of sexual behavior.* New York: Raven Press.

Dieckmann, G., & Hassler, R. (1975). Unilateral hypothalamotomy in sexual delinquents: Report on 6 cases. *Confinia Neurologica, 37,* 177-186.

Doerr, P., Kockott, G., Bogt, H. H., Pirke, K. M., & Dittmar, F. (1973). Plasma testosterone, estradiol and semen analysis in male homosexuals. *Archives of General Psychiatry, 29*(6), 829-833.

Doerr, P., Pirke, K. M., Kockott, G., & Dittmar, F. (1976). Further studies on sex hormones in male homosexuals. *Archives of General Psychiatry, 33,* 611-614.

Dörner, G. (1968). Hormonal induction and prevention of female homosexuality. *Journal of Endocrinology, 42,* 163-164.

Dörner, G. (1979). Hormones and sexual differentiation of the brain. In *Sex, hormones and behaviour.* Ciba Foundation Symposium, *62.* Amsterdam: Excerpta Medica.

Dörner, G. (1974). Sex hormone dependent brain differentiation and sexual functions. In G. Dörner (Ed.), *Endocrinology of sex: Differentiation and neuroendocrine regulation of the hypothalamo-hypophysial-gonadal system.* Leipzip: Johann Ambrosius Barth.

Dörner, G., Geier, T., Ahrens, L., Krell, L. Münx, G., Sieler, H., Kittner, E., & Müller, H. (1980). Prenatal stress as a possible aetiogenetic factor of homosexuality in human males. *Endokrinologie, 75*(3), 365-368.

Dörner, G., & Hinz, G. (1968). Induction and prevention of male homosexuality by androgen. *Journal of Endocrinology, 40,* 387-388.

Dörner, G., Rohde, W., Seidel, K., Haas, W., & Schott, G. (1976). On the evocability of a positive oestrogen feedback action on LH secretion in transsexual men and women. *Endokrinologie, 67*(1), 20-25.

Dörner, G., Rohde, W., Stahl, T., Krell, L., & Masius, W. (1975). A neuroendocrine predisposition for homosexuality. *Archives of Sexual Behavior, 4*(1), 1-8.

Ehrhardt, A. A., Epstein, R., & Money, J. (1968). Fetal androgens and female gender identity in the early-treated andrenogenital syndrome. *Johns Hopkins Medical Journal, 122*(3), 160-167.

Ehrhardt, A. A., Evers, D., & Money, J. (1968). Influence of androgen and some aspects of sexually-dimorphic behavior in women with the late-treated adrenogenital syndrome. *Johns Hopkins Medical Journal, 123*(3), 115-122.

Ehrhardt, A. A., & Meyer-Bahlburg, H. F. L. (1981, March) Effects of prenatal sex hormones on gender-related behavior. *Science, 211,* pp. 1312-1318.

Eisinger, A. J., Huntsman, R. G., Lord, L., Merry, J., Polani, P., Tanner, J. M., Whitehouse, R. H., & Griffiths, P. D. (1972). Female homosexuality. *Nature, 283,* 106.

Evans, R. B. (1972). Physical and biochemical characteristics of homosexual men. *Journal of Consulting and Clinical Psychology, 39*(1), 140-147.

Foucault, M. (1978). *The history of sexuality. Volume I: An introduction* (R. Hurley, Trans.). New York: Random House.

Freud, S. (1961). *Drei Abhandlungen zur Sexualtheorie.* In *Gesammelte Werke,* Fünfter Band, pp. 29-145. London: Imago Publishing. (Originally published, 1905).

Freud, S. (1975). [Three essays on the theory of sexuality] (J. Strachey, Trans. & Ed.). New York: Basic Books. (Originally published, 1905)

Friedman, R. C., Dyenfurth, I., Linkie, D., Tendler, R., & Fleiss, J. L. (1977). Hormones and sexual orientation in men. *American Journal of Psychiatry, 134*(5), 571-572.

Gadpaille, W. (1980). Biological factors in the development of human sexual identity. *Psychiatric Clinics of North America, 3*(1), 3-20.

Gartrell, N. K. (1982). Hormones and homosexuality. In W. Paul, J. D. Weinrich, J. C. Gonsiorek, & M. E. Hotvedt (Eds.), *Homosexuality: Social, psychological and biological issues.* Beverly Hills, CA: Sage.

Gartrell, N. K., Loriaux, D. L., & Chase, T. N. (1977). Plasma testosterone in homosexual and heterosexual women. *American Journal of Psychiatry, 134*(10), 1117-1119.

Glass, S. J., Deuel, H. J., & Wright, C. A. (1940). Sex hormone studies in male homosexuality. *Endocrinology, 26*(4), 590-594.

Glass, S. J., & Johnson, R. W. (1944). Limitations and complications of organotherapy in male homosexuality. *Journal of Clinical Endocrinology, 4*(10), 540-544.

Goy, R. W., & McEwen, B. S. (1980). *Sexual differentiation of the brain: Based on a work session of the Neurosciences Research Program.* Cambridge, MA: Massachusetts Institute of Technology Press.

Griffiths, P. D., Merry, J., Browning, M. C. K., Eisinger, A. J., Huntsman, R. G., Lord, E. J. A., Polani, P. E., Tanner, J. M., & Whitehouse, R. H. (1974). Homosexual women: An endocrine and psychological study. *Journal of Endocrinology, 63,* 549-556.

Herron, R. (1981). Born gay. Review of *Sexual preference: Its development in men and women* by A. P. Bell, M. S. Weinberg, & S. K. Hammersmith. *Christopher Street, 59,* 55-57.

Hines, M. (1982). Prenatal gonadal hormones and sex differences in human behavior. *Psychological Bulletin, 92*(1), 56–80.

Jaffee, W. L., McCormack, W. M., & Vaitukaitis, J. L. (1980). Plasma hormones and the sexual preference of men. *Psychoneuroendocrinology, 5*(1), 33–38.

Kennedy, H. C. (1980/81). The "Third Sex" theory of Karl Heinrich Ulrichs. *Journal of Homosexuality, 6*(1/2), 103–111.

Kenyon, F. E. (1974). Female homosexuality: A review. In J. A. Loraine (Ed.), *Understanding homosexuality: Its biological and psychological bases.* New York: American Elsevier.

Kinsey, A. C. (1941). Homosexuality: Criteria for a hormonal explanation of the homosexual. *Journal of Clinical Endocrinology, 1*(5), 424–428.

Kolodny, R. C., Jacobs, L. S., Masters, W. H., Toro, G., & Daughaday, W. H. (1972). Plasma gonodotropins and prolactin in male homosexuals. *Lancet, 2,* 18–20.

Kolodny, R. C., Masters, W. H., Hendryx, J., & Toro, G. (1971). Plasma testosterone and semen analysis in male homosexuals. *New England Journal of Medicine, 285*(21), 1170–1174.

Kolodny, R. C., Masters, W. H., Kolodner, R. M., & Toro, G. (1974). Depression of plasma testosterone after chronic intensive marijuana use. *New England Journal of Medicine, 290*(16), 872–874.

Krafft-Ebing, R. von. (1950/1939). *Psychopathia sexualis: A medico-forensic study.* New York: Pioneer Publications (Translation of German twelfth edition, originally published, 1886).

Kreuz, L. E., Rose, R. M., & Jennings, J. R. (1972). Suppression of plasma testosterone levels and psychological stress. *Archives of General Psychiatry, 26, 479–482.*

Kulin, H. E., & Reiter, E. O. (1976). Gonadotropin and testosterone measurements after estrogen administration to adult men, prepubertal and pubertal boys, and men with hypogonadotropism: Evidence for maturation of positive feeback in the male. *Pediatric Research, 10,* 46–51.

Laughlin, H. (1914). *The legal, legislative and administrative aspects of sterilization.* Report of the committee to study and to report on the best practical means of cutting off the defective germplasm in the American population. Cold Spring Harbor, Long Island, NY: Eugenics Record Office Bulletin No. 10B.

Lauritsen, J., & Thorstad, D. (1974). *The early homosexual rights movement.* New York: Times Change Press.

Lev-Ran, A. (1974). Sexuality and educational levels of women with late-treated adrenogenital syndrome. *Archives of Sexual Behavior, 3*(1), 27–32.

Livingstone, I. R., Sagel, J., Distiller, L. A., Morley, J., & Katz, M. (1978). The effect of luteinizing hormone releasing hormone (LHRH) on pituitary gonadotropins in male homosexuals. *Hormone and Metabolic Research, 10,* 248–249.

MacCulloch, M. (1980). Biological aspects of homosexuality. *Journal of Medical Ethics, 6,* 133–138.

MacCulloch, M., & Waddington, J. L. (1981). Neuroendocrine mechanisms and the aetiology of male and female homosexuality. *British Journal of Psychiatry, 139,* 341–345.

MacLusky, N. J., & Naftolin, F. (1981, March 20). Sexual differentiation of the central nervous system. *Science, 211,* 1294–1303.

Masica, D. N., Money, J., & Ehrhardt, A. A. (1971). Fetal feminization and female gender identity in the testicular feminizing syndrome of androgen insensitivity. *Archives of Sexual Behavior, 1*(2), 131–142.

Meyer-Bahlburg, H. F. L. (1977). Sex hormones and male homosexuality in comparative perspective. *Archives of Sexual Behavior, 6*(4), 297–325.

Meyer-Bahlburg, H. F. L. (1979). Sex hormones and female homosexuality: A critical examination. *Archives of Sexual Behavior, 8*(2), 101–119.

Money, J. (1980). *Love and love sickness: The science of sex, gender differences, and pair-bonding.* Baltimore: The Johns Hopkins University Press.

Money, J., & Dalery, J. (1976). Iatrogenic homosexuality: Gender identity in seven 46,XX chromosomal females with hyperadrenocortical hermaphroditism born with a penis, three reared as boys, four reared as girls. *Journal of Homosexuality, 1,* 357–371.

Money, J., & Mathews, D. (1982). Prenatal exposure to virilizing progestins: An adult follow-up study of twelve women. *Archives of Sexual Behavior, 11*(1), 73–83.

Money, J., & Ogunro, C. (1974). Behavioral sexology: Ten cases of genetic male intersexuality with impaired prenatal and pubertal androgenization. *Archives of Sexual Behavior, 3*(3), 181–205.

Money, J., & Schwartz, M. (1977). Dating, romantic and nonromantic friendships, and sexuality in 17 early-treated adrenogenital females, aged 16–25. In P. A. Lee, L. P. Plotnick, A. A. Kowarski, & C. J. Migeon (Eds.), *Congenital adrenal hyperplasia*. Baltimore, MD: University Park Press.

Müller, D., Orthner, H., Roeder, F., König, A., Bosse, K., & Kloos, G. (1974). Einfluss von Hypothälamusläsionen auf Sexualverhalten und gonadotrope Funktion beim Menschen. Bericht über 23 Fälle. [Influence of hypothalamic lesions on sexual behavior and gonadotropic function in men: A report of 23 cases.] In G. Dörner (Ed.), *Endocrinology of sex*. Leipzig: Johann Ambrosius Barth.

Nieschlag, E. (1979). The endocrine function of the human testis in regard to sexuality. In *Sex, hormones and behaviour*, Ciba Foundation Symposium, *62*. Amsterdam: Excerpta Medica.

Noble, R. G. (1979). Male hamsters display female sexual responses. *Hormones and Behavior, 12*, 293–298.

Parks, G. A., Korth-Schutz, S., Penny, R., Hilding, R. F., Dumars, K. W., Frasier, S. D., & New, M. I. (1974). Variation in pituitary-gonadal function in adolescent male homosexuals and heterosexuals. *Journal of Clinical Endocrinology and Metabolism, 39*(4), 796–801.

Perkins, M. W. (1981). Female homosexuality and body build. *Archives of Sexual Behavior, 10*(4), 337–345.

Perloff, W. H. (1949). Role of the hormones in human sexuality. *Psychosomatic Medicine, 11*, 133–139.

Pillard, R. C., Rose, R. M., & Sherwood, M. (1974). Plasma testosterone levels in homosexual men. *Archives of Sexual Behavior, 3*(5), 453–458.

Pirke, K. (1974). Psychosexual stimulation and plasma testosterone in men. *Archives of Sexual Behavior, 3*, 577–584.

Rohde, W., Stahl, F., & Dörner, G. (1977). Plasma basal levels of FSH, LH and testosterone in homosexual men. *Endokrinologie, 70*(3), 241–248.

Rose, R. M. (1978). Neuroendocrine correlates of sexual and aggressive behavior in humans. In M. A. Lipton, A. DiMascio, & K. F. Killiam (Eds.), *Psychopharmacology: A generation of progress*. New York: Raven Press.

Rosenzweig, S., & Hoskins, R. G. (1941). A note on the ineffectualness of sex-hormone medication in a case of pronounced homosexuality. *Psychosomatic Medicine, 3*(1), 87–89.

Sand, K., & Okkels, H. (1938). The histological variability of the testis from normal and sexual-abnormal, castrated men. *Endokrinologie, 19*(6), 369–374.

Sigusch, V., Schorsch, E., Dannecker, M., & Schmidt, G. (1982). Official statement by the German Society for Sex Research (Deutsche Gesellschaft für Sexualforschung e. V.) on the research of Prof. Dr. Günter Dörner on the subject of homosexuality. *Archives of Sexual Behavior, 11*(5), 445–449.

Stahl, R., Dörner, G., Ahrens, L., & Graudenz, W. (1976). Significantly decreased apparently free testosterone levels in plasma of male homosexuals. *Endokrinologie, 68*(1), 115–117.

Starka, L., Sipova, I., & Hynie, J. (1975). Plasma testosterone in male transsexuals and homosexuals. *Journal of Sex Research, 11*(2), 134–138.

Tourney, G., & Hatfield, L. M. (1973). Androgen metabolism in schizophrenics, homosexuals and normal controls. *Biological Psychiatry, 6*(1), 23–36.

Tourney, G., Petrilli, A. J., & Hatfield, L. M. (1975). Hormonal relationships in homosexual men. *American Journal of Psychiatry, 132*(3), 288–290.

Ulrichs, K. H. (1975) *Forschungen über das Rätsel der mannmännlichen Liebe, 12* volumes in one. New York: Arno Press. (Originally published, 1898)

VanLook, P. F. A., Hunter, W. M., Corker, C. S., & Baird, D. T. (1977). Failure of positive feedback in normal men and subjects with testicular feminization. *Clinical Endocrinology, 7*, 353–366.

Wooden, W. S., & Parker, J. (1982). *Men behind bars: Sexual exploitation in prison*. New York: Plenum Press.

Yalom, I. D., Green, R., & Fisk, N. (1973). Prenatal exposure to female hormones. *Archives of General Psychiatry, 28*(4), 554–561.

BOOK REVIEWS

PAEDOPHILIA: THE RADICAL CASE. Tom O'Carroll. *London: Peter Owen, 1980, pp. 280.*

ADULT SEXUAL INTEREST IN CHILDREN. Mark Cook and Kevin Howells, editors. *London (and New York): Academic Press, 1981, pp. xii+275.*

The year 1977 seems to have been an *annus mirabilis* for the study of pedophilia and related issues: the year of Boston's indictment of 24 suspected pederasts (Note 1) and the resultant formation of the Boston-Boise Committee as a publicly active political group for pederasts (Mitzel, 1980); the year of the House Committee on the Judiciary, Subcommittee on Crime hearings into the sexual exploitation of children (Committee on the Judiciary, 1977); and the year of the seminal International Conference on Love and Attraction at Swansea, England, under the auspices of the British Psychological Society (Cook & Wilson, 1979). Mark Cook was an organizer of the Swansea conference, Kevin Howells convened a symposium on Pedophilia, and Tom O'Carroll, at the time of the conference Chairperson of the Pedophile Information Exchange (PIE) in London, attended on behalf of his organization. After a gestation period of some three years, these three men, in separate efforts, gave us the two books reviewed here, books which show every indication that the subject of pedophilia will never be the same as it was before 1977.

Tom O'Carroll's book is plainly a political manifesto which, through remarkable objectivity and understanding of many issues outside his self-stated expertise, leads to an indictment of current sex-repressive social customs with the suggestion that age-of-consent laws and other restrictions on child sensuality/sexuality be abolished. The Cook/Howells volume is number 22 in the publisher's "Personality and Psychology" series, and contains nine papers by eleven authors, some of whom are established scholars in the study of pedophilia and other modes of sexuality, and at least four of whom were present at the 1977 Swansea Conference. That the efforts resulting in these two books, while not collaborative, were interrelated is documented in each work by a description of the conference and its importance to O'Carroll and to Cook and Howells. For Tom O'Carroll the Conference on Love and Attraction was one of several places chosen as vehicles to enter PIE's philosophy, indeed its very existence, into the British press and hence into the nation's consciousness; the result was ultimately disastrous, as O'Carroll describes in detail in his Chapter 12. Indeed, as Cook and Howells report in their preface, the potential for disaster stalked the conference as a whole, mostly in the "person" of PIE, the presence of which caused a public reaction "so strong . . . that the conference came very close to being cancelled" (Cook and Howells, p. vii), though these editors strongly infer that this public reaction was at least part of the catalyst which led them to begin "planning this book with the intention of assembling a body of information about the various aspects of adult sexual interest in children, which might provide a factual basis for a cooler and more reasoned approach to the issue" (p. viii). Further evidence of commonality between the two books is found in the fact that editor Kevin Howells and several of the authors in the Cook/Howells book are referenced by O'Carroll, and conversely, an article by O'Carroll is referenced (Chapter 8, p. 243) by Kenneth Plummer in the Cook/Howells collection.

Tom O'Carroll faced the presumably difficult problem of his own credibility as a pedophile writing a book about pedophilia in a clear and comprehensive statement (Chapter 1) outlining his personal development, "first loves" and other experiences, his teaching career and the aftermath of his dismissal for a non-sexual attachment to an eleven-year-old boy. We become acutely aware at the very beginning that here is a man whose principles are important to him, and who refuses to capitulate to an authority which will not acknowledge his style of loving, even if it means losing his career and prestige in the community. His accounts of his reasoning, his actions and his reactions lay the foundation for understanding both the "how" and "why" of so concerted and exhaustive a research effort as the one he presents in the rest of his book.

And research it is, though the author as an educator-writer, not a scientist, clearly understands and states his limitations, for he brings together a wide range of writings in psychology, sociology, radical politics, literature, anthropology and elsewhere to document his points. Opinions are carefully labeled and both sides of an issue consistently are presented as prelude to the author's argument of his own position. This, along with the logical structure of the book from definitions through descriptions of the participants and the nature of pedophilic acts to legal reform based on the needs and rights of children and other issues, gives the book a definite respectability which is not dependent on the reader's agreement with the conclusions reached by the author.

As may be expected, O'Carroll's assumptions cannot be said to be proven by the literature assembled on their behalf; indeed, there are few if any points in the social sciences which can be "proven." Among the assumptions is the author's belief that, like the homosexual who was once thought to be pathological, the pedophile represents a different orientation which is not necessarily sick, but whose manifest problems are often due to the pressures imposed by a less-than-understanding society. Also, the child is seen as a sexual being with both capacity for and tendency toward genital contact, though such contact represents a different experience for the child than for the adult (just as in Piagetian theory the child's cognitive structures are different from those of the adult). Sex is assumed to be harmless *per se,* with observed trauma due primarily to the reactions of important adults in the child's life. These assumptions, and others, lead to the central proposition of the book, that the whole "problem" of pedophilia is really a problem of a sex-repressive society ignoring—or rather crashing up against—the reality that expression of sexuality is natural in some form for all persons at all stages of life.

Given a situation where natural inclinations (on the part of both children and pedophiles) are being frustrated, where "inalienable rights," if you will, are being denied with often cruel results to "victims" of all ages, the author feels justified in demanding radical action to rectify the situation as he sees it. He offers, in the form of PIE's platform, extensive and detailed suggestions for law reform based on the concept of "willingness" to participate in non-harmful activities, rather than the more restrictive and problematical idea of "informed consent." This is possible, he asserts, without resorting to an arbitrary "age of consent" so long as the child has a reliable way out of the situation and is taught that it is proper in some situations to say "no" to adults. This would be enforced by civil, not criminal, courts where no force or physical harm is involved and parents would be able to intervene, up to a point, on behalf of the child. Though the temptation might be to see this approach as one of the weak points of the book, one is continually reminded that the radical perspective requires that the situation be restructured in all its aspects, leaving potential critics in the position of speculating, like the author himself, rather than knowing what would happen in such situations. Hence, if children were raised in an atmosphere of sexual freedom without the consequences of such actions as we know them today, perhaps they would be considered "qualified" at any age to make their own sexual decisions.

But what of the question of power inequality between child and adult? The author addresses this issue with comparisons to other situations in which a child needs or wants something and an adult does or does not provide it, and *vice versa.* His argument is that power differentials exist in every child-adult contact, whether it be schooling, parenting or other nonsexual sharing of affection, and while there is always the "*potential* for abuse" (p. 167, author's italics), more often than not the inequality of power works to the advantage of the child's development. Since "healthy" pedophilic relationships would arise only where the child has needs/desires which the pedophile wishes to fulfill, power differentials would become an issue only in coercive relationships and could be handled as such under the civil/legal structure proposed earlier (Chapter 6).

Paedophilia: The Radical Case accomplishes its purposes: it delineates and clarifies the issues surrounding pedophilia and sexuality in general; it offers alternatives both of sweeping attitudinal and social reforms and minutely specific legal changes; it assesses current social trends and marks the path from the present to the author's proposed future solutions; and it manages to document the issues and proposed changes with literature from varying disciplines while at the same time maintaining the humanistic approach characteristic of an involved and caring person who wants not to destroy but to create and contribute.

That the author sometimes sounds idealistic, or approaches unrealistic optimism, should be viewed in context, for he never loses sight of his underlying principle: "the vision is not merely the narrow one 'pedophile liberation', but of liberating the *positive* potential that resides in everyone's body" (p. 248, author's emphasis). The main criticism likely will be that O'Carroll is not qualified to analyze critically the research he cites, though he does attempt to provide the interdisciplinary approach heretofore missing in pedophilia studies. That the author is not a professional (a "scientist", if you will) is typical of the study of *verboten* topics; however, now that the ground is broken it becomes the task of the research community to fill the void.

The first step toward filling this void may very well exist in *Adult Sexual Interest in Children*. This collection of nine articles deals, in separate sections, with (1) Children, (2) Adults, (3) Assessment and Treatment and (4) The Wider Context (i.e., pedophilia in society). Each article is either a report of original research, a contribution to a theoretical structure, a proposal of action or possible future research, or a combination of these approaches. A common problem of past research on pedophilia is continued here, in that almost all data reported were gathered from pedophiles in therapy, in prison, or both, making generalizations to the total pedophile population ill-advised; however, this problem is clearly recognized by the editors and most of the authors, and their suggestions for future research include an awareness of the need for studies of non-patient and non-prison subjects. Almost every author raises the issue of emotionality surrounding the question of pedophilia, and firmly states her/his/their intention to remain as objective as possible. This, combined with the consistent use of value-neutral terminology in place of emotion-laden terms such as "molestation," "abuse," "perverted" or "abnormal," represents a definite departure from almost all previous literature dealing with child-adult sexual contact.

Chapter 1 presents a literature review which seeks to delineate the differences and similarities between physical abuse and sexual abuse of children as it occurs within families only. Various types of literature are considered separately (e.g., psychological, cultural studies, psychosocial) and analyzed as to the characteristics of the subjects studied and the dynamics of the individuals and groups described. Regarding the source of physical abuse as compared with sexual abuse, the authors found less difference than similarity, which was surprising to them considering the fact that the two types of abuse are usually treated separately in the literature. While this article provides potentially useful distinctions between types of abuse, causes, precipitating factors and high-risk family and parental types, the conclusions rest on the results of other studies and are restricted to the dynamics and situations found within families; these two limitations tend to restrict the applicability of the conclusions to sexually or physically abusive situations occurring outside a family setting. Authors of Chapter 1 were Constance Avery-Clark, Joyce Ann O'Neil and D. R. Laws, all associated with Atascadero State Hospital (maximum security mental facility dealing with sex offenders and others) in California.

In Chapter 2, J. W. Mohr distills from his previous work a variety of information regarding the relationship of age to various aspects of pedophilia, including the age distribution of the adults and of the children involved in such contacts, and findings regarding the average age of sex objects and types of behavior characteristic of each of the three distinct groups of offenders studied: namely, the adolescent (average age about 15), middle adult (average age around 35) and older adult (average age around 55). It is unfortunate that this short article offers nothing more than a paragraph regarding the age characteristics associated with male children, as most data describe female children in heterosexual pedophilic contacts. Despite the tantalizing brevity of the discussion of age structures, the author makes a strong case in his introduction and throughout for future consideration of pedophilia in non-judgmental terms, regarding sexuality in children realistically and honestly, and questioning the popular assumption that pedophilia is necessarily deviant, an assumption which traditionally has biased pedophilia research to the point of uselessness.

Kevin Howells, in Chapter 3, reviews the development of the literature dealing with psychological aetiology of pedophilia in the psycho-analytical and "social learning" schools of thought, discusses the important considerations in future formulation of theories regarding pedophilia, and cautions against drawing conclusions about aetiology from biased samples of pedophiles. As the author notes, attempts at aetiological theory have been limited in scope and based on small samples of non-representative subjects; his review covers the time since Freud, but appropriately concentrates on recent literature. While his review of the pedophilia literature is not comprehensive, the points of his article solidly are underscored: pedophilia is represented in many types of people and acts, rather than being a single, simple condition; and research in pedophilia must delineate the types of people, acts, motivations and other components of the issue before aetiology can be attempted.

Chapter 4 presents an overview by Thore Langfeldt (University of Oslo, Norway) of the history, process (physical and social) and content (behavioral and attitudinal) of sexuality development in children. While a reading of the article gives one the feeling that a fresh, unbiased approach is providing a more realistic picture of a once-taboo subject, the critical reader will notice the lack of substantiating references which leaves one unable to determine whether the knowledge comes from the author's reading, his observations, experimental work or a combination of these.

Chapter 5 consists of data from original articles by the author, Matti Virkkunen, augmented by additional similar studies which view the child's behavior as a significant part of the interaction in a pedophilic contact. The understandable logic is that without the child's participation the act could not occur and certainly could not continue into a relationship, unless it involved force (which most pedophilic acts do not). This contribution is valuable in its illumination of just what the pedophilic act can and does mean to the child: the child most likely sees the act less in sexual terms than does the adult, viewing it rather as exciting in a more general way, a way of receiving attention, or a way of relating with adults socially. The article is limited in that it discusses only female children in heterosexual pedophilia.

Kurt Freund in Chapter 6, drawing on his extensive background in the assessment of sexual (or erotic) response in humans, discusses the various techniques of assessing arousal (e.g., phallometric, chemical) and the relationship of arousal to erotic interest, including detailed descriptions of procedures and equipment as well as clear and original definitions of the components of sexual arousal in humans. This is followed with a short section on the application of these techniques and concepts to pedophilia and a comment on the use of phallometry in therapeutic experimentation as a measurement of the effects of therapy in eliminating or altering patterns of erotic arousal. Though the article borders precariously on the assumption that pedophilic impulses are automatically improper and need redirection (an assumption not supported by any evidence in his article and one which other authors in this volume have avoided), the author never states this position and actually offers information about techniques which could be useful to researchers studying, among other topics, the extent of pedophilic responses in the general population.

David A. Crawford's contribution in Chapter 7 deals with treatment of pedophiles, including irreversible treatments such as castration and certain anti-libidinal drugs, and more humane approaches such as psychotherapy, behavior modification, and skills training to name a few. Though the article is based on an assumption that sex offenders *ipso facto* are in need of some sort of treatment, if for no other reason than they are socially anomalous, the author acknowledges the controversy regarding treatment of sexual deviance in the very first sentence of his article, and properly states that such considerations of propriety are outside the scope of his paper. He aims his survey of the literature, concepts, techniques in use and future directions, toward "individuals who are genuinely seeking help and are as disturbed by their own behavior as is the rest of society" (p. 182).

In Chapter 8, Kenneth Plummer offers his perspective on constructing a sociological baseline for the study of pedophilia. His intent is to apply to pedophilia principles developed within the "sociology of deviance" (p. 221) and thereby to suggest future directions for pedophilia research. This is a theoretical article which takes advantage of the implied freedom to draw on the collected wisdom of his discipline and extrapolate. While purists might wish for a more research-based approach—regardless of the fact that this is currently impossible—the intent here is to provide as wide an overview as possible and establish a framework which will help researchers and more pedantic theorists understand the larger picture, from the point of view of the author, before they attempt to support or refute the finer points. Plummer investigates the stereotypes involved in pedophilia, and presents opposing positions which tend to emphasize the humanness of pedophiles; he investigates pathology arguments and points out that they are not based on data, but rather on the unipolar assumption that pedophiles are sick; he discusses the view that pedophilia is deviant and points out that to some all non-procreative sex is deviant, making pedophilia's deviance merely a matter of degree in the value structure of the "beholder," as it were; and finally, he discusses the position of the pedophile in the social/psychological systems of society in which he (pedophiles are usually males) is perceived as a threat mainly because of society's one-dimensional, distorted understanding of him.

The concluding Chapter 9, by D. J. West, author of *Homosexuality* (1960, 1968) and *Homosexuality Re-examined* (1977), provides the author's insights into possible methods of dealing with adult sexual interest in children in the future. His well-taken point is that recent research, including the studies of the present volume reviewed here, does not always provide complete understanding of the causes of the problem and direct routes to solutions, for "questions are raised and complexities discovered that had never been thought of before" (p. 251). He suggests further research in several specific areas using existing and innovative techniques, and does so through a careful and systematic analysis of the issues and problems associated with the incidence of pedophilia, child sexuality, adult offenders and the acts they become involved in. His general approach to social control, as he puts it, is one of decreased punitive and increased rehabilitative measures, including centers where pedophiles may present themselves for help without fear of punishment; relaxed attitudes in society toward sex, especially child sexuality and sex education; and a serious reconsideration of the appropriateness of age-of-consent laws, when sufficient laws against force and coercion also exist.

With the publication of these volumes, then, it is abundantly clear that "all the past is (but) prologue" in research dealing with pedophilia, and that the entire field well may be re-evaluated beginning now. Formed in the same conference at Swansea and proceeding from different orientations, these books raise issues, problems and questions which illustrate clearly the possibility, feasibility, even inevitability, of revised public attitudes and renewed interest in research.

Gerald Jones, PhD (cand.)

REFERENCE NOTE

1. The term "pederasts" is used to distinguish these men, who were involved with younger males, from men whose attraction is to younger females or youngsters of both sexes. The distinction is arbitrary, however, and the more general term "pedophile" is also used in this review, as it was the term used in the original books.

REFERENCES

Committee on the Judiciary, House of Representatives. (1977). *Sexual exploitation of children.* Washington, DC: U.S. Government Printing Office.

Cook, M., & Wilson, G. (1979). *Love and attraction: An international conference.* Oxford: Pergamon Press.

Mitzel, J. (1980). *The Boston sex scandal.* Boston: Glad Day Books.

West, D. J. (1968). *Homosexuality.* 2nd ed. Harmondsworth, Middlesex: Penguin. (originally published, 1960)

West, D. J. (1977). *Homosexuality re-examined.* London: Duckworth.

Index

abortion 30,37*n*.
Adult Sexual Interest in Children (Cook and
    Howells) 95,98–102
affection
  interpersonal 15,39
  reciprocal 17,18,21–22,23,24
aggression 41
American Psychological Association 31
androgens
  in animal models 70,71
  deficiency 70,77
  as homosexuality treatment 72
  in sex differentiation 69,70,71,77
anima muliebris 67
animal models, of homosexuality 68–71,83
  androgen effects 70,71
  extrapolation to human behavior 70–71,
    83–85
  mating behavior 68–70
  sexually dimorphic behavior 68–69,71,76,
    85
arousal-cue response
  definition 15
  DSM-III classification 16
  in exhibitionism 24
  in homosexuality 20
  reciprocal affection and 22
  in sadomasochism 18,19
asphyxiophilia 23

bestiality, *see* zoophilia
biological factors, *see also* genetic factors;
    hormonal factors
  in bisexuality 84–85
  in heterosexuality 86–87
  in homosexuality
    prenatal brain differentiation 66,67,
      69–71,76–82
    sexual dimorphism 68–69,71,76,85
    stress 77
biological sex 15
bisexuality
  biological factors 84–85
  hormonal factors 78
  occurrence 41
brain, prenatal sex differentiation in 76–82
  in animal models 69–71
  hormonal factors 70–82
  Ulrich's theory of 66–67

children, *see also* pedophilia
  homosexual identity 7,8
  sexual development 6
congenital adrenal hyperplasia 79–80,82
consciousness-raising therapy 43,46,47–49
constructionist therapy 39–51
  case examples 43–50
  consciousness-raising 43,46,47–49
  definition 40
  essentialist concepts and 40–50
    clinician's response to 42–50
    false consciousness 43,47
    homosexuals' attitudes 42–43
    limitations 41
    role theory 42
    therapeutic implications 40
    transsexualism 41–42,47–49,50
coprophilia 10
cross-dressing, *see* transvestism

Diagnostic and Statistical Manual, sexual
    disorder classifications 9–28
  arousal-cue response patterns 16,18,19,20
  fantasy as criterion 15,17–18,19
  homosexuality
    ego-dystonic 9,11–14,21
    moral considerations 32–33,34–35
    mental disorder concept 11–13,20–21
  paraphilias 10,14–26,33,34–35
    moral considerations 33,34–35
    as psychological disorders 19–21
    social mores and 10,26

ego dystonias
  homosexuality 9,11–14,21,62
  as mental disorders 21
estrogen, in sex differentiation 69,70,71
  in animal models 70,71
  feedback mechanism 77–78,79
exhibitionism
  diagnostic criteria 15,17,24
  DSM-III classification 9–10,14,24
  fantasy in 18
  reciprocal affection in 18
  research on 20
experimentation 56

fantasy, paraphiliac 15,16–17,18,19,20
fellatio 57

    103

For Product Safety Concerns and Information please contact our EU representative GPSR@taylorandfrancis.com Taylor & Francis Verlag GmbH, Kaufingerstraße 24, 80331 München, Germany

T - #0141 - 270225 - C0 - 229/152/10 - PB - 9780918393012 - Gloss Lamination